Medicine
by Design

ARCHITECTURE, LANDSCAPE, AND AMERICAN CULTURE SERIES
Katherine Solomonson, University of Minnesota—Series Editor

Medicine by Design: The Architect and the Modern Hospital, 1893–1943
ANNMARIE ADAMS

The Architecture of Madness: Insane Asylums in the United States
CARLA YANNI

A Manufactured Wilderness: Summer Camps and the Shaping of American Youth, 1890–1960
ABIGAIL A. VAN SLYCK

Medicine by Design

The Architect and the Modern Hospital, 1893–1943

ANNMARIE ADAMS

UNIVERSITY OF MINNESOTA PRESS

MINNEAPOLIS • LONDON

Material from chapter 2 was previously published in Cheryl Krasnick Warsh and Veronica Strong-Boag, eds., *Children's Health Issues in Historical Perspective* (Waterloo, Ontario: Wilfrid Laurier University Press, 2005). An earlier version of chapter 2 appeared as Annmarie Adams and David Theodore, "Designing for 'The Little Convalescents': Children's Hospitals in Toronto and Montreal, 1875–2006," *Canadian Bulletin of Medical History* 19, no. 1 (2002): 201–43; reprinted with permission. A shortened version of chapter 3 appeared in Gail Dubrow and Jennifer Goodman, eds., *Restoring Women's History through Historic Preservation* (Baltimore: The Johns Hopkins University Press, 2003). An earlier version of chapter 3 appeared as "Rooms of Their Own: The Nurses' Residences at Montréal's Royal Victoria Hospital," *Material Culture Review* (formerly *Material History Review*) 40 (Fall 1994): 29–41; reprinted with permission. An earlier version of chapter 5 was previously published as "Modernism and Medicine: The Hospitals of Stevens and Lee, 1916–1932," *Journal of the Society of Architectural Historians* 58, no. 1 (March 1999): 42–61; reprinted with permission.

Published by the University of Minnesota Press
111 Third Avenue South, Suite 290
Minneapolis, MN 55401-2520
http://www.upress.umn.edu

Printed in the United States of America on acid-free paper

Library of Congress Cataloging-in-Publication Data

Adams, Annmarie.
  Medicine by design : the architect and the modern hospital, 1893-1943 / Annmarie Adams.
     p. ; cm. — (Architecture, landscape, and American culture series)
  Chapters previously published in various books and journals.
  Includes bibliographical references and index.
  ISBN: 978-0-8166-5113-9 (hc : alk. paper)
  ISBN-10: 0-8166-5113-2 (hc : alk. paper)
  ISBN: 978-0-8166-5114-6 (pbk. : alk. paper)
  ISBN-10: 0-8166-5114-0 (pbk. : alk. paper)
  1. Hospital architecture—North America—History. 2. Hospital buildings—
Design and construction—North America—History. I. Title. II. Series.
  [DNLM: 1. Hospital Design and Construction—trends—Canada—Collected Works.
2. History, 19th Century—Canada—Collected Works. 3. History, 20th Century—
Canada—Collected Works. WX 140 A211m 2008]
  RA967.A33 2008
  725'.51—dc22
                                                    2007038121

The University of Minnesota is an equal-opportunity educator and employer.

15 14 13 12 11 10 09 08   10 9 8 7 6 5 4 3 2 1

IN MEMORY OF

John William Adams

1924–2004

Contents

Illustrations

Acknowledgments

I have many individuals and institutions to thank for their help with this book. First and foremost, I am grateful to David Theodore, a skilled researcher and discerning reader. The evolution of the project was driven by countless inspirational conversations with him about the nature of architectural research, and many of the insights presented here are his.

A number of other graduates of McGill's School of Architecture also contributed to the project. Céline Lemercier gathered materials at Hôpital Notre Dame, Hôpital Ste-Justine, and the Sir Mortimer B. Davis Jewish General Hospital of Montreal. James Clark undertook a useful photographic history of the Royal Victoria Hospital in fall 2000. Nadia Meratla and David Theodore cocurated the exhibition "Hospital Architecture: Treasures from McGill's Collections" in 1999, which uncovered new material and inspired fresh ways to consider the sources. François-Xavier Caron secured permissions for the illustrations.

This project benefited from generous internal and external financial support. The research began with a modest Seed Grant for Faculty Research in 1993 from the McGill Centre for Research and Teaching on Women, to study the nurses' residences at the Royal Victoria, still the core of chapter 3. I later received two grants from the Hannah Institute for the History of Medicine in 1994 and 1997, which covered the costs of collecting general material on Stevens and Lee. Fonds pour la formation des chercheurs et d'aide à la recherche also supported the project with a three-year grant from their program for *nouveaux chercheurs* (1994).

A new project on Canadian hospitals since World War II, supported by the Canadian Institutes of Health Research in the form of a Health Career Award (2000–2005), along with a Social Sciences and Humanities Research Council of Canada and three more Hannah grants, provided indirect and direct benefits to this earlier work by allowing me to continue to support a team of dedicated McGill students and by subsidizing smaller-scale projects, such as an ongoing initiative to construct a virtual history of Canadian hospitals and a project on spatial responses to tuberculosis in Montreal. Central to the success of these ongoing projects were Hrant Boghossian, LeeAnn Croft, Víctor Garzón, Solange Guaida, Valerie Minnett, Jan Schotte, Peter Sealy, and Ricardo Vera.

Hospital administrators are often reluctant to expose their historical documents to architectural historians. This is particularly likely if (1) the material is unsorted or (2) the future of the building is threatened. Most of the hospitals included in this book satisfied both these conditions, and yet their administrators cooperated fully in the interests of historical research. I express my deep gratitude to all the hospital staff members who opened their unedited vaults, basements, and closets to us. There are too many individuals to mention, but special thanks go to Pat Blanshay, the late Martin Entin, and the late Brenda Cornell at the Royal Victoria Hospital; Christopher Rutty for his help on the Connaught Laboratories; R. Peter Thompson at the Ottawa Civic Hospital; William Feindel at the Montreal Neurological Institute; and Jack Charters at the Montreal Children's Hospital.

As an institution particularly proud of its medical heritage, McGill University has archives and libraries extremely rich in documents pertaining to hospital history. I would like to acknowledge the committed staffs of the McGill University Archives, the Osler Library of the History of Medicine, the Life Sciences Library, the Rare Books and Special Collections Division, the John Bland Canadian Architecture Collection, and the Blackader-Lauterman Library for help with this research over many, many years. Librarian Marilyn Berger secured a grant of her own to document hospital resources in Montreal in 2000, which served to raise awareness of hospital design among students and Montrealers. Daniella Rohan and Julie Korman of the John Bland Canadian Architecture Collection discovered and conserved nearly fifty original drawings by Henry Saxon Snell, which became the heart of chapter 1. Former chief curator of rare books Irena Murray supported this project in numerous ways.

Christian Paquin permitted me to photograph his outstanding collection of postcards of Montreal hospitals, which has served as a unique source of evidence both in the book and as a way to study the evolving form of the typology, particularly the Royal Victoria Hospital. The Canadian Centre for Architecture, too, is an invaluable resource, especially the library's outstanding collection of early-twentieth-century journals.

My friends and colleagues at the School of Architecture at McGill University have supported this project in myriad ways, from tolerating piles, overflowing boxes, and gigantic rolls of dusty old blueprints outside my office, to granting me a sabbatical year in 2000 to work on the book. For their ongoing interest in this work I especially thank Ricardo L. Castro, David Covo, Derek Drummond, Helen Dyer, David Krawitz, Robert Mellin, the late Norbert Schoenauer, Pieter Sijpkes, and Radoslav Zuk. Students at McGill heard far too many versions of this research in my courses over the past decade; I thank them now for never complaining.

Many other people lent their expertise to the project at various stages. Deserving special mention are Philip Cercone, Jim Connor, Gail Dubrow, Raphael Fischler, Paul

Groth, Cynthia Hammond, Margaretta Lovell, Tania Martin, Sherry Olson, Mary Anne Poutanen, Thomas Schlich, Kevin Schwartzman, and Dell Upton. David Sloane, Kate Solomonson, Abby Van Slyck, and two anonymous reviewers read the manuscript and made suggestions that greatly improved the book.

Peter Gossage is a model scholar and editor, and he has participated in every detail of this project. The younger members of our family also played active roles in this research. Friends have joked at the lengths I was willing to go to undertake primary-source research at the Royal Victoria Hospital: during the course of working on this book I gave birth there twice, to Charlie in 1996 and to Katie in 1999. *Medicine by Design* is lovingly dedicated to their grandfather, Jack Adams, a champion of hospital improvement, who died suddenly before this book was finished.

Introduction

My personal interest in twentieth-century hospital design comes from imagining a history of medicine from built sources, rather than relying solely on written texts. My doctoral research had touched on this challenge through an analysis of women, doctors, and late-nineteenth-century house design. Hospitals seemed like a logical next step from the healthy house. Were hospitals catalysts in the development of modern medicine? Or were they, as many architectural and medical historians had assumed, simply passive reflections of medical innovation? The sheer volume of buildings constructed between the wars, too, demanded scholarly attention. The 1920s saw an enormous growth in the numbers of hospitals constructed.[1] In Montreal, for example, the number of hospital beds actually doubled during this time.

About the time of World War I a fundamental revolution in the design of generic medical space occurred, too.[2] The Royal Victoria Hospital in Montreal, not far from my office at McGill University's School of Architecture, is a stunning illustration of this change. Designed by British architect Henry Saxon Snell in 1889–93, the original "Royal Vic" was a typical pavilion-plan building. Snell and others believed that the large open wards and the isolation of patients with particular diseases into separate pavilions discouraged the spread of infection. In its H- or E-shaped massing, the pavilion-plan hospital looked like a prison, school, convent, or other large institution associated with social reform. Surveillance, light, and fresh air were the central ideas. Stopping the spread of infection was its central intention.

American architects Edward F. Stevens and Frederick Lee's additions to the Royal Vic in 1916 and 1925 represented a completely different approach to the hospital plan. The Ross Memorial Pavilion and Montreal Royal Victoria Maternity Hospital, built overlooking Snell's sprawling, neo-Scottish Baronial hospital, were examples of the so-called block plan, which was more compact than the earlier pavilion concept. Stevens and Lee designed an arrangement of smaller patient rooms along double-loaded corridors to encourage contact among medical specialists, but couched their efficient plans in castlelike exteriors. Aristocratic homes and luxurious hotels provided the inspiration for the architecture of the interwar hospital block, upstaging the references to prisons and schools preferred by Snell. Healing patients was its central intention.

Historians of architecture and medicine frequently explain this transformation from the pavilion plan to the block plan with reference to the germ theory, particularly to Robert Koch's discovery in the 1870s that specific bacilli caused particular diseases. This suggestion that the germ theory meant the end of the pavilion-plan hospital is unconvincing on several counts. Pavilion-plan hospitals continued to be built into the 1930s, at the same time as block-plan buildings.[3] Besides, the explanation is counterintuitive. The discovery that germs, rather than bad air, spread disease might make an open ward even more effective, rather than obsolete.

Architectural historian Adrian Forty has suggested that the eclipse of the pavilion plan resulted from a diminished confidence on the part of the medical profession in hospital buildings as "instruments of cure," and a move to increase investment in medical technology. Forty also argues that patients had more and more influence over hospital design as wealthier patients were attracted to the institution. In general, like this study, Forty refutes the argument put forward by historians of medicine that advances in medical technology change hospital form. His warning that the "lack of any clear causal relationship between scientific discovery and innovation in building form suggests that more attention should be given to the motives of those who controlled hospitals than to the development of science" inspired the writing of this book.[4]

Sociologist Lindsay Prior, on the other hand, believes that more attention should be paid to the social context of hospital design. "The acceptance of germ theory found its initial expression in the siting and design of the operating theater and the laboratory, but from there it moved outward and into the wards," he writes, emphasizing the design as a passive receptor of medical innovation. "The architecture of hospitals is, therefore, inextricably bound up with the forms of medical theorizing and medical practice which were operant at the hour of their construction and, what is more, all subsequent modifications to hospital design can be seen as a product of alterations in medical discourse," Prior claims. Much of his argument was presumably aimed at Nikolaus Pevsner, who had suggested that hospital design was the product of architects' creativity.[5]

In perhaps the most direct attempt to analyze medical buildings as artifacts of medical history, historian J. T. H. Connor has illustrated how particular spaces, like the operating room, or building types, like the general hospital, the asylum, or even the physician's office, can illuminate significant stages in the history of medicine. Although this may be obvious to historians of art and architecture, it is an approach rarely employed by historians of medicine.[6] They more typically use buildings as illustrations, privileging, instead, written sources on their particular subject. Connor noted this pattern in his much-cited 1990 review essay, "Hospital History in Canada and the United States," in which he suggested that the use of images of hospitals on the covers of hospital histories implied that the texts were concerned with architecture, while they typically were not. In this essay—

another inspiration for this project—Connor also underlined the need for synthetic studies of hospitals in Canada.[7]

Connor's concern about buildings as passive sources in the history of medicine inspired me to reconsider the hospital's image. As an architectural historian, I knew the decades of the 1920s and 1930s as the golden age of Modernism, marked by the construction of International Style buildings like Le Corbusier's Villa Savoye in Poissy, France.[8] Hospitals of the interwar period were more likely to resemble Georgian mansions or Italian palazzos than the revolutionary, machinelike forms that I showed to students in my introductory courses on architectural history. In terms of architectural style, Stevens and Lee's additions to the Royal Victoria looked a lot like Snell's earlier hospital. In fact, today's visitors to the hospital still have trouble telling the original and subsequent sections apart, demonstrated by the complex system of letter-based signage devised by the hospital to orient staff and visitors. Just how and where did architecture and medicine intersect in the arrangement of the general hospital? And how did physicians and architects work together to modernize the hospital?

METHODOLOGY

As the book's title is intended to suggest, *Medicine by Design* is about the complex teams of experts and users who made the early-twentieth-century hospital. It is a case study approach to a single building type. Particular places and institutions in this study, particularly the Royal Victoria Hospital in Montreal, and recognized experts, such as Stevens and Lee, defined the state of the art in hospital design. But the buildings they produced were typical, not exceptional. Indeed, the Royal Victoria Hospital and its subsequent additions appear again and again in this book because an in-depth look at a single place over time allowed me to track the dynamic relationship of architecture and medicine.[9] The hospital's opening date, 1893, provides the starting point of the book and the focus of its first chapter, because it marked a significant moment in the history of Canadian hospital architecture.[10] And the building has remained, since that time, the site of avant-garde medical space and expertise. The Royal Victoria is Canada's premier example of the pavilion-plan type and its subsequent architecture is a panorama of architectural forms, including the dignified edifices of the interwar decades, the bold, undecorated towers of the 1960s, and the high-tech, patient-centered facilities of the 1990s. It was the site of influential additions by significant international hospital architects. In addition to Snell and Stevens and Lee, whose buildings are discussed extensively in this study, the Royal Victoria Hospital commissioned other world-class, nonspecialist architects to work on its physical plant. The Olmsted firm produced a landscape plan in 1896 that was never realized.[11] McKim, Mead & White, of New York, repaired the main facade of the building in 1907. A list of local architects who had a hand in its pre–World War II design reads like a Who's Who of Canadian architectural history: J. W. Hopkins, Andrew Taylor, Hutchison and Wood, Edward and W. S. Maxwell, Nobbs

& Hyde, Ross & Macdonald, and Lawson & Little. This coterie of important international and local architects is evidence of how the Royal Victoria Hospital's design has
stood the test of time, remaining authoritative even after its ideals became obsolete.

A major contribution of the study is that it outlines how architects played an active role
in the development of twentieth-century medicine and how doctors played an active
role in the development of twentieth-century architecture. My argument is not that interwar hospital architecture was therapeutically efficacious, but rather that it anticipated and
produced medical practices broadly and socially conceived, rather than just reflected them
symbolically. Similarly, the juxtaposition of patients, nurses, physicians, and architects in
the chapter titles expresses the reciprocal significance of architecture and medicine for
each other as interactive factors in the evolution of the twentieth-century hospital.

A second important contribution of the book is that it bridges the subfields of elite
and vernacular architecture studies. Dell Upton's book on Virginia churches, Abigail
Van Slyck's studies of Carnegie libraries and summer camps, and Elizabeth Cromley's
research on New York apartment buildings are the models for this hybrid, experiential
approach to an architectural typology.[12]

The time period covered in this book comes from the cohort of case studies. The
construction of the Royal Victoria in 1893 opened a distinct era in the history of Canadian hospital architecture, and the retirement of Edward F. Stevens in 1943 marked
the brink of a completely different chapter in the institution's design in North America
and Europe. Hospitals after Stevens (and coincidentally, after World War II) were mostly
bold, undecorated towers, like those at the postwar Royal Vic, with little connection to
their regional architectural traditions.

Even in the 1940s, critics suggested that architectural design was only a passive reflec-
tion of medical change. James Marston Fitch included only one hospital illustration in
his classic 1947 survey of architecture in the United States. The caption accompanying
the photograph of the Lake County Tuberculosis Sanatorium of Waukegan, Illinois,
designed by Ganster and Pereira, is a typical expression of this assumed causal relationship of medicine and architecture in the scholarly literature. "Advances in medicine
are brilliantly paced by the glass walls and southern balconies of Ganster and Pereira's
hospital at Waukegan, Ill.," the caption reads, suggesting that the building can barely keep
up with changes in tuberculosis treatment.[13] By 1947, however, the use of fresh air and
sunlight as treatments for tuberculosis was a century old. What advances in medicine did
the hospital "pace"?

An essential aspect of my research methodology was to explore hospitals in the context of other building types. A host of nineteenth-century institutions in which large
groups of people were housed (and transformed in some way) resembled hospitals in
plan, section, and elevation. Prison and orphanage plans allowed guards and matrons
to survey their charges at a glance, just like nurses watched over their patients in the
pavilion-plan ward. School and hospital architects used classical details and symmetrical
planning to bestow their institutions with a dignified community presence. Convent and

hospital design, at least in Montreal, showcased new technologies for heating and lighting long before they appeared in houses. And hotels, like private patients' hospitals constructed in the 1920s and 1930s, offered travelers the utmost in luxury and refinement as a form of entertainment, relaxation, and desire. Even industrial building types, notably factories, presented to the designers of hospital kitchens new ways of assembling, cooking, and distributing food to patients in bed. And the great halls of train stations, I believe, were the inspiration for massive hospital waiting rooms in outpatient clinics.

Linking architectural spaces to everyday hospital activities such as meal preparation and waiting to see a doctor is an equally important aspect of my approach to the hospital in this book. As institutions that never close and are thus in constant motion, hospitals are ideal buildings in which to study use. For years my dream has been to stumble upon a source that documents how an individual might have moved through hospital space. The best I've ever found are the accounts I use in chapter 2, which I engage to suggest that rich and poor patients moved through the hospital in fundamentally different ways. Wealthy patients experienced the hospital in a smooth, uninterrupted movement, often entering the building at the level of an upper floor from an automobile; poorer patients, on the other hand, sometimes entered through the basement, directly from the streetcar stop, and experienced the general hospital in jarring, sporadic movements. This finding has already made me eager to study how social class and gender affect movement in other building types, such as hotels or train stations. How can we know?

The modernized hospital also offered an irresistible opportunity to explore how architectural ideas transgress or perhaps ignore national boundaries. Decades before the North American Free Trade Agreement took effect in 1994, the careers of architects such as Stevens played across the Canadian-U.S. border. Even since NAFTA, remarkably few architectural histories have explored the notion of a North American architectural narrative.[14] Why not?

Finally, a substantial part of approaching hospitals as artifacts of material culture is taking a closer look at the stuff inside them (furniture, finishes, technologies, everything) than is usually the case in architectural history. The design and placement of radiators, blanket warmers, elevators, acoustical insulation, and bedside tables serve as evidence in this story of the sometimes tense, always interesting relationship of architecture and medicine.

The initial project to study the change from the pavilion-plan to the block-plan hospital quickly outgrew the Royal Vic. This growth in scope occurred in two significant directions. First, the investigation was enlarged to include all general hospitals constructed in Montreal between the wars. A team of students visited these hospitals and gathered the relevant documents: architectural drawings, photos, descriptions, newspaper reports, board minutes, and any other sources related to hospital design. Second, an attempt was made to locate these hospitals within the burgeoning constellation of hospital specialists. Stevens and Lee were prolific designers of hospitals in the early twentieth century and had constructed the two aforementioned significant additions to the Royal Vic in the interwar period: the Ross Memorial Pavilion and the Montreal Royal Victoria Maternity Hospital. Their names appear over and over again in conjunction with other hospital expansions, in both Canada and the United States. Since the partnership designed more than one hundred prominent institutions in its practice (which ran from 1912 to 1933), the firm is a reliable gauge of trends in hospital design during an important time in hospital reform. And given that Stevens began to specialize in hospitals in the 1890s, his career spanned the exact half century under study.

Another reason for turning to Stevens as a focus for the project was that unlike most busy twentieth-century architects, he wrote about his firm's work. Stevens's book, *The American Hospital of the Twentieth Century*, is a classic analysis of modern hospital planning. Because there are no extant archives of the firm, the buildings were forced to speak for themselves. Printed sources notwithstanding, this material-culture approach to the buildings allowed us to test whether architecture and artifacts tell different stories than do printed sources in the history of medicine.[15] The project expanded to consider as many Stevens and Lee projects as I could reasonably visit. Stevens's book and his hundreds of published journal articles, of course, were invaluable sources on the rest of his oeuvre, including hospitals as far away as Peru.

STYLE

Interpreting the social history of the built environment means considering architectural style mostly as a tool used by hospital architects, rather than a category of analysis. Stevens's perspective on architectural style was complex. He considered his hospitals to be forward-looking, despite their multiple references to historic styles. This situation was not unique to hospital design. Office towers, public buildings, churches, schools, libraries, and even houses that appear stylistically traditional were considered modern by those who designed, produced, sponsored, or used them.[16]

Associating with local architectural firms was one way that Stevens tried to soften the impact of new hospital buildings. He and his colleagues believed that the place-based knowledge of generalist architects trumped his specialized knowledge of hospitals with no particular geographic focus when it came to the design of the hospital's image. Specialists like Stevens might point to the hospital's structure, its endorsement of aseptic medical practice, its sanctioning of expert knowledge, its appeal to new patrons, its encouragement of new ways of working, its response to urbanization, its use of zoning, its acceptance of modern social structures, its resemblance to innovative building types, its embrace of internationalism, and its endorsement of standardization, as evidence of its so-called Modernism. To the doctors who worked in them, Stevens's hospitals offered the latest medical and nonmedical technologies, including surgical suites, underground tunnels, and car parking. To patients, the new hospitals boasted luxurious quarters, a call system for nurses, in-house dining, and a fabulous view over the older, outdated hospital and the industrial city.

Indeed, to specialists like Stevens a historical or locally inspired style was a way in which he modernized the hospital. Until the 1940s, good health was related to traditional values, through the symbols of home associated with traditional architecture, such as pitched roofs, classical entries, interior molding, masonry construction, and discrete rooms. Hospitals, in fact, relied on the likeness of the big, safe house to convince middle-class city dwellers that their chances were as good there as they were at home, especially to those who might pay much-needed extra fees for semiprivate or private accommodation, as we will see in chapter 2, or to young middle-class women interested in becoming professional nurses, as discussed in chapter 3. This marketing of the remade institution as a modern one may have been the intention of a photograph of the superintendent of Hôpital Notre-Dame (Figure I.1), who likely rearranged his office so that the perspective of the Stevens-designed building would appear in the image, just like his telephone, metal filing cabinet, and his other trappings associated with a forward-looking workplace.

A brief look at the other major hospitals in Montreal operating in 1893 illustrates these priorities and allegiances. By the time the Royal Vic opened, the Hôtel-Dieu, an

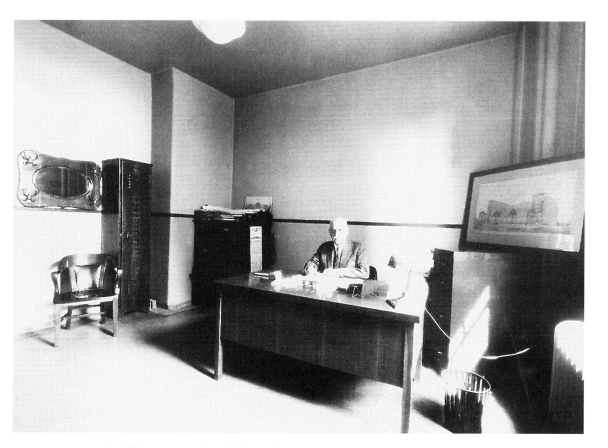

FIGURE I.1. The superintendent of Hôpital Notre-Dame, circa 1930, surrounded by the trappings of the modern office, including an architectural perspective.

institution founded in the seventeenth century, occupied a monumental building at the corner of Pine and St. Urbain streets designed by Victor Bourgeau. By then the monumental cruciform-plan building had undergone relatively few additions (only the construction of a dwelling for the chaplain and a dispensary in 1886). At its center was a monumental chapel. The western half of the building accommodated the sisters (Religieuses Hospitalières de Saint-Joseph), while the hospital was located in the institution's east wing. Like many classically planned institutions, the Hôtel-Dieu occupied a walled site, including extensive gardens. Its identity as a Roman Catholic hospital is underscored in section and elevation by the chapel's magnificent dome and axial entry sequence, rather than in its arrangement of medical spaces.

The city's second major Catholic hospital is a good illustration of the tensions between French-speaking institutions. Founded in 1880 by a branch of the Laval Medical Faculty who had been excluded from the Hôtel-Dieu, Notre-Dame was run by the Montreal School of Medicine and Surgery. Like the Royal Vic, Notre-Dame declared itself blind to ethnic and religious differences: "devoted to the poor and unfortunate sick of all races and creeds."[17] Like many Victorian institutions, it had an early history of occupying renovated buildings.[18]

The Montreal General Hospital (MGH), too, occupied a series of sites before the opening of its first purpose-built edifice, accommodating seventy-two patients, on May 1, 1822. An image of 1826, the first known sketch of the hospital, shows the building as a rectangular, three-story, five-bay block, with a shallow hipped roof and classical cupola (which illuminated its first operating room), as designed by Thomas Phillips. The central entry is raised and arched; the windows in this central bay are also larger than the others, and arched; the corners of the building are decorated with quoins. This early hospital is set back from the street, surrounded by one-story gabled buildings and an iron fence, and accessible through an arched gateway. The *Hochelaga Depicta* (1839) shows the building in 1831, after the addition of the Richardson wing. In 1848, the Reid wing was built; to the rear of the Reid wing was added the Morland wing, for children, in 1874. Just a year before the opening of the Royal Victoria, the MGH saw the opening of two surgical pavilions and a large operating theater; at the same time, Montreal architect Andrew Taylor remodeled the old building for medical, gynecological, and ophthalmic patients. It boasted electricity and telephones; its nursing school opened in 1890 (the building was erected in 1897).

Religion, as a spatial determinant of hospital design, has been accorded too much importance in our understanding of Montreal hospital and institutional architecture. W. D. Lighthall began the section on charitable and religious buildings in his 1892 guidebook to the city, *Montreal after 250 Years*, by noting "the sharp division of Roman Catholic and Protestant hospitals," qualifying his remark, however, by adding that "the charity of some of the institutions is broader than their denominational limits."[19] I would only add to Lighthall's footnote that the architecture of these institutions, too, extended beyond religious boundaries, a nuance difficult to read in written sources.

The Outline of This Book

In an attempt to understand hospital buildings as artifacts of material culture, *Medicine by Design* is composed of five thematic essays, rather than a chronology of hospital design. The first and fourth chapters deal most directly with the architectural features of the hospital. Chapter 1 focuses on the architectural form of the hospital at the end of the nineteenth century. "1893" attempts a synchronic snapshot of one typical late-nineteenth-century hospital. By looking at the design intentions of its famous architect and what was actually built, chapter 1 shows how hospital architecture was fiercely contested and, by implication, how buildings are dynamic products of widely varying ideals. The approach engaged in this first chapter—a close reading of architectural drawings and related documents to assess how various theories or cultural priorities can be traced in the built environment—is useful for the study of other typologies and time periods. Here sources include unbuilt or partly built hospital designs, photographs, letters, annual reports, city guidebooks, and newspapers. Chapter 1 is a starting point from which four issues are subsequently explored, each in its own chapter: (1) international expertise, (2) social class, (3) gender, and (4) modernism.

The book turns in chapters 2 and 3 to the users of the modern institution, examining the hospital through the lenses of social class and gender. New patient groups accommodated in the institution of the 1920s are the subject of chapter 2: paying patients, outpatients, women, and children. Chapter 3 brings us back again to the site of the Royal Victoria Hospital, where we observe in detail how changes in the spaces intended for nurses reveal their changing role in the increasingly complex institution.

Chapter 4, "Architects and Doctors," examines the rising tensions between twentieth-century hospital experts. This discussion focuses on a general overview of the buildings designed by Edward Stevens but also includes the international scope of his career as architect, prolific author, and influential hospital expert. Chapter 5, "Modernisms," outlines a series of new architectural features legible in hospitals designed during or after World War I. I argue that Stevens and Lee, and other hospital architects of their era, clothed modern hospital plans in regionally inspired imagery in order to smooth the effects of social and medical change taking place within the walls of the institution. These five thematic essays, ranging in focus from architectural intentions to user experience, attempt to capture the dynamic, complex relationships of the North American hospital, its makers, and its users over a half century.

The chapters work in concert to show that interwar hospital architecture did not simply reflect medical innovation. Rather, architects, health-care experts, and users worked in a dynamic alliance to produce a building typology that was simultaneously futuristic and reactionary; highly specialized and generic; distracting and peaceful. Hospital architects looked to homes, hotels, and other building types for inspiration, and what resulted was a complex, hybrid, and dignified institution.

1893

In 1893, Montreal was a deeply layered city. Framed by the mighty St. Lawrence River and picturesque Mount Royal, the city from a distance appeared as a dense, sloping grid of tiny, attached houses. Monumental, gable-roofed churches with towers and bulky religious and educational institutions, especially monasteries and convents, punctuated the layer of flat-roofed houses and provided clear visual hierarchies in the mostly Catholic, French-speaking metropolis.[1] So, too, did the splendid commercial structures of the early twentieth century. A 1906 panoramic view of the city showcases the city's commercial growth from the old city at the river's edge, toward the mountain (Figure 1.1). Sophisticated

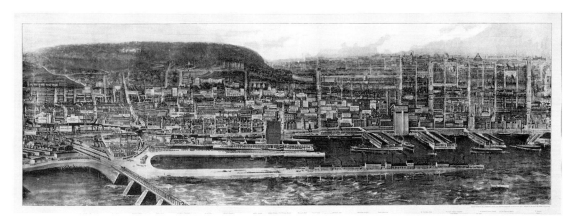

FIGURE 1.1. Panoramic view, "Montreal A.D. MDCCCCVI."

commercial buildings—banks, hotels, insurance companies, and department stores—expressed the immense industrial wealth that built late-nineteenth-century Montreal and underscored the social and linguistic divisions that layered the city's complex physical structure.

This remarkable panorama also documents the Royal Victoria Hospital, hovering ghostlike against the backdrop of Mount Royal. Like the church towers, convents, and businesses of Montreal, its architecture emphasized horizontal layering and vertical separation. First conceived in honor of Queen Victoria's Golden Jubilee in 1887 as a charitable institution for the poor, the Royal Vic provided a general response to disease. Accommodating its patients in large, open wards, the Royal Vic was a modified H-plan, with a five-story central administration block and two long, narrow wings facing south.[2] Owing to the steepness of the site, the first floor of the western ward (surgical) was level with the third floor of the eastern ward (medical), lending the ensemble a serrated, asymmetrical silhouette. Slender, cylindrical towers anchored the southern corners of the rectangular wards, accommodating sanitary facilities for its 250 patients, who were separated by illness, gender, and age, depending on the space available at any given time.[3]

The hospital's terraced, grassy courtyard was broken only by a circular driveway and by paths leading beneath rather minimal stone bridges connecting the administration block and the wards. Elegant cast-iron sun porches graced the narrow ends of the surgical and medical wards, between the towers, and were arranged to catch the southern exposure and the magnificent views of the city, the St. Lawrence River, and apparently even Vermont on clear days.

Directly south of the new hospital was McGill University. By 1893, the campus included a dozen or so freestanding limestone (known in Montreal as "greystone") buildings with pitched copper roofs, loosely grouped around a long, straight driveway leading up from Sherbrooke Street, the northern boundary of the city's growing commercial district. Most notable among these buildings was the Arts Building, a neo-Palladian masterpiece designed by John Ostell in 1839–43, whose outstretched eastern and western wings welcomed visitors to the institution. The Redpath Museum of 1882 and Redpath Library of 1893, just to the west of the axial entry, were showcases of the university's architectural allegiances to Scotland. To the west of McGill, mostly along Sherbrooke Street and Pine Avenue, the busy thoroughfare that separated the university from the Royal Vic, stretched Montreal's famous Square Mile. The area's sumptuous mansions and New York–style apartment blocks accommodated 70 percent of Canada's wealth by 1900.[4]

To the southeast of the hospital lay the area now known as the McGill Ghetto, a dense residential district of duplexes and triplexes that housed lower-middle-class Montrealers before its transformation to a popular student neighborhood in the late twentieth century. As mentioned earlier, the city's commercial core, including modern department stores, office buildings, and elegant squares, lay south of Sherbrooke Street. Directly to the northwest of McGill, and central to the genesis of the Royal Vic, was the city's municipal water reservoir.

A much-reproduced postcard of the time (Figure 1.2) shows the south side of Pine Avenue fenced by a rather primitive wooden palisade. Montrealers "of all races and creeds without distinction, and mainly of those who are in indigent circumstances" arrived at the hospital by foot or by horse-drawn carriage, past a tiny polygonal gatehouse that marked the entrance to the site from the busy, steeply sloped, urban thoroughfare.[5]

The Royal Vic on its opening day, December 2, 1893, offers us a unique opportunity to explore the character of typical hospital design immediately preceding the major period of focus in this book, setting the stage for the four subsequent chapters. How were debates concerning ideal hospital design borne out in real architecture in the late nineteenth century? Who were hospital experts, and how was their expertise developed and assessed? I engage visual evidence in order to tease out how changes in medical theory can be read in the built environment. In particular, what do extant architectural drawings say about the designer's intentions, and how does the hospital as constructed speak of the forces that required him to compromise those ideals?

From a single case study at a particular moment, Montreal's Royal Victoria Hospital in 1893, we glean a plethora of information on a range of topics: the multifunctional role of hospitals in the city, the significance of hospital location, the hospital as a philanthropic enterprise, the role of architects as hospital specialists, the development of hospital typologies (in this case, the pavilion plan) as a coherent subgroup of buildings, and the ward and its surrounding hospital as a healing technology. The architecture of

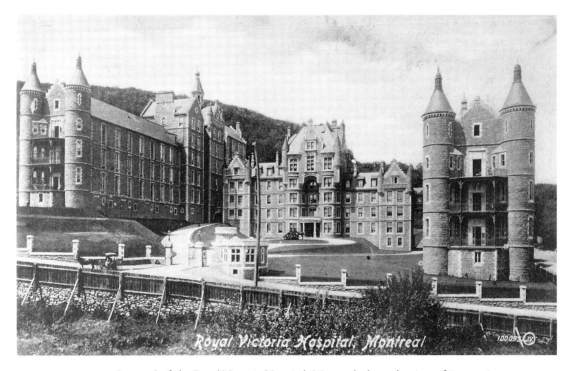

FIGURE 1.2. Postcard of the Royal Victoria Hospital, Montreal, about the time of its opening.

surgery, design for ventilation and isolation, and the provision of staff quarters are discussed in depth, as these parts of the hospital become the focus of significant reforms in the ensuing decades.

Hospital as Civic Monument

An important characteristic of the Royal Vic was that its civic function complemented its everyday use as a hospital. The original building was an astonishing success as both a monument and a tourist attraction, even before it opened for patients. Admirers of the building typically pointed to its mountainside site. "The Victoria Hospital, though new, stands at the head of all," reported W. D. Lighthall in his 1892 guidebook to the city, *Montreal after 250 Years;* "it dominates the city from the top of University Street."[6] Its location on the southern slopes of Mount Royal, a prominent wooded 223-meter mountain (developed into a vast urban park by Frederick Law Olmsted and inaugurated in 1876) is key to this impression of urban domination by the hospital. Mount Royal not only inspired the city's name but also figures prominently in its foundation story as the site where French explorer Jacques Cartier was guided by the people of the village of Hochelaga in 1535. Today the mountain holds a 31.4-meter illuminated cross, installed in 1924, which symbolizes the Roman Catholic background of most French-speaking Montrealers.

The hospital's magnificence was appreciated for decades after its opening. Even after World War I, the Royal Victoria Hospital was still a favorite among authors of guidebooks to the city: "the beauty of its site, the excellence of its management, and the cleverness of its doctors have given this institution a fame that reaches out far beyond the confines of Montreal," attested Charles W. Stokes, author of *Here and There in Montreal,* in 1924.[7] The hospital's distinction as a tourist site is underlined by its difference from other hospitals at the time. Despite their inclusion in popular guidebooks, not all pre–World War II Montreal hospitals were popular tourist attractions. The convent hospitals and especially the Hôtel-Dieu, while decidedly monumental buildings, were apparently too religious for most tourists. Lighthall described the Grey Nuns' hospital as one of "monastic vastness and severity of outline," while Stokes admitted only that the Hôtel-Dieu was "not unhandsome."[8] And the more secular hospitals—the Montreal General of 1821, the Western of the 1880s, and Hôpital Notre-Dame of the 1880s—were not especially impressive as built, although they still sometimes were mentioned in guidebooks. The Montreal Board of Trade's 1893 semicentennial report, in fact, included photographs of the Montreal General Hospital, the Hôtel-Dieu, and the Royal Victoria. And other hospitals did appear on postcards, such as Hôpital Notre-Dame and the Western General Hospital (Figures 1.3 and 1.4).

But until World War II, only the Royal Victoria was an immediate and lasting success as both monument and landmark.[9] In addition to its highly visible location, this success derived from the building's sheer scale, its picturesque configuration, its association

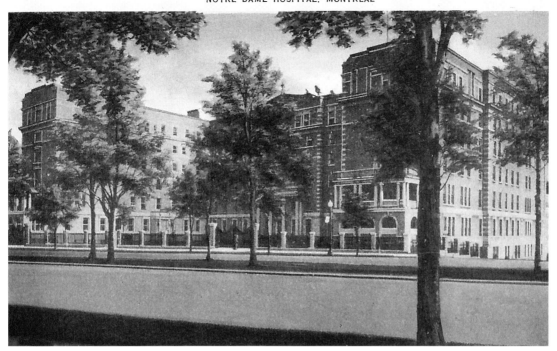

FIGURE 1.3. Postcard of Hôpital Notre-Dame, Montreal.

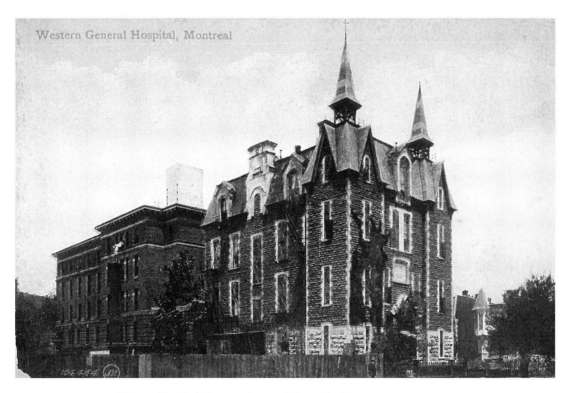

FIGURE 1.4. Western Hospital, Atwater Avenue, Montreal, circa 1900.

(through the pavilion-plan typology) with the extent of the British Empire, and its romantic, Scottish baronial detailing. Montreal photographer William Notman produced a superb series of photographs of the hospital in 1894. His firm's potent images had already contributed to the success of many other tourist attractions, including the construction of the Grand Trunk and Canadian Pacific Railways, and Montreal's remarkable Victoria Bridge of 1858.[10] These achievements, like the hospital, were technological wonders of their time, and Notman's photos helped to make them famous.

The press of the 1890s certainly anticipated the new hospital with awe. "In appointments and general arrangements, it will have no rival in its particular sphere of usefulness on the continent of America," reported one of the city's English-language dailies, the *Gazette*, in 1891, more than two years before the hospital's opening.[11] Journalists generally equated the institution's novelty with specific architectural features and details, such as the sophisticated set of multiple entries to the hospital, as well as the ways particular building materials were handled. The spacious lobby, featuring a statue of Queen Victoria seated with two young children on the first landing of a graceful, bifurcated wooden stairway, was considered particularly elegant. As patients were not permitted to enter the administration block, this gracious entryway was mostly for seventy-five paid staff and board members, whose dedicated spaces surrounded the hospital's main entry on all levels.[12] Patients were intended to drive under the bridge linking the west ward and the central block, entering the administration building on the west side of its third floor.[13] Snell's longitudinal cross section (Figure 1.5) of the hospital illustrates the minimal links between the administration block and the wards, which were essentially short bridges located on the third floor. Apart from these two connections, each block of the tripartite Royal Victoria was basically freestanding. And the wards, it was said, would have no corners, in order to avoid the accumulation of dust. In addition to these more general features, the reporter also noted the technical prowess of the design: elevators, fireproofing, easy-to-inspect drainage pipes, and electricity.

Location, Location, Location

The location of the new hospital was significant beyond its symbolism. By 1893, preferred sites for urban hospitals across North America were distant from the noise and pollution of the industrial city; Mount Royal offered the opportunity to raise the hospital, both symbolically and physically, above the streets and buildings of Montreal. "The situation is unequalled, and cannot but be of great benefit in every way to the sick," claimed the author of the *Official Guide and Souvenir* for the British Medical Association's conference in Montreal. "Standing as it does, isolated, and on the brow of the Mountain, facing the south, there is abundance of light and air."[14]

The building's status as a civic monument was likely augmented by the intense debates surrounding its location, especially given that the City of Montreal contributed the land for the new building in 1887. Next to the grandiose Hugh Allan estate, both its proximity to the existing municipal water reservoir and its distance from the city center worried physicians.[15] The donors then purchased land from the Frothingham estate, just to the east of the city site, in order to extend the plot to University Street. Provided the hospital itself would be built on this extension, a little farther from the reservoir, the extended site was considered acceptable.

Guidebook authors directed tourists to the hospital on account of its beauty. The Royal Vic was described as "the handsomest in the city" by no less than the Master Painters' and Decorators' Association of Canada in 1904, in the souvenir guide to Montreal they published for their first convention, held at the city's elegant Windsor Hotel.[16]

Philanthropy

Although popular as a civic monument, the hospital in 1893, it must be remembered, was essentially an institution for the poor. Canadians who could afford it paid for medical care at home, at least until after World War I. Until that time, those wholly or partially

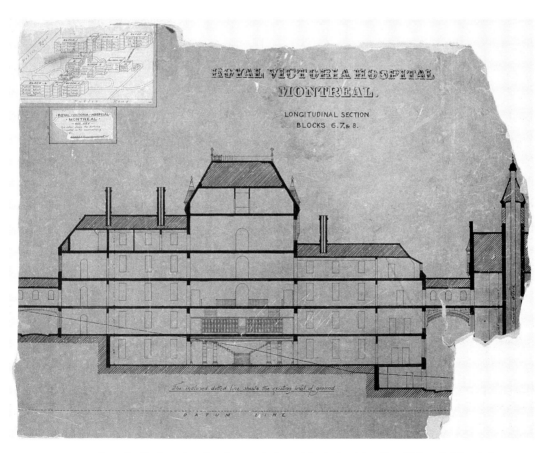

FIGURE 1.5. Longitudinal section showing vertical spatial relationships, Royal Victoria Hospital.

unable to cover the costs of medical treatment for themselves could be admitted to a general hospital. Recommendations from a board member or clergy were not even necessary for admission. Potential patients could simply apply in person at the hospital, or a house doctor might arrive at a patient's home in an ambulance to transport him or her there. Services were provided by a combination of voluntary support, municipal grants, and private donations.[17]

Not surprisingly given this level of accessibility, the Royal Victoria Hospital's first annual report (1894) indicates a range of patients and outcomes. The administration reported admitting "1570 patients; of these 1345 were discharged, 776 cured, 401 improved, 97 unimproved, 71 not treated, 84 died, and 141 remained." These first patients were 861 males, 709 females; 1,017 Protestants, 501 Catholics, 52 other religions. At 29.3 days, the average stay per patient in 1894 at the Royal Victoria Hospital was extremely long relative to today's standards.[18]

The hospital's convenience too came from its premise as a "castle" for the poor, made possible through the generosity of two of Canada's wealthiest industrialists, Donald Smith and George Stephen. Born in Scotland, these cousins dominated the Montreal anglophone business establishment. About the time of the hospital's founding, Smith was governor of the Hudson's Bay Company, the oldest and most storied commercial enterprise in Canada. He also founded the Royal Victoria College for women at McGill University in 1896, whose elegant building designed by Bruce Price defined the southeast corner of the campus. Stephen is credited with the success of the Canadian Pacific Railway, serving as its first president from 1880 to 1888. Both men were elevated to the peerage. Smith became first Baron Strathcona and Mount Royal in 1897, while Stephen was made a baronet in 1886, and became first Baron Mount Stephen in 1891. Both Smith and Stephen returned to England at the end of their careers; Smith was High Commissioner for Canada in England until his death in 1914. Stephen in particular was a generous benefactor to many institutions and is reported to have given away more than $1 million during his lifetime.

The Expert Architect

A third, lesser-known figure in the genesis of the Royal Victoria Hospital as a civic monument is its designer, London-based architect Henry Saxon Snell (1830–1904). He was well known throughout the English-speaking world as the author of two influential texts on hospital architecture, *Hospital Construction and Management* (1883), which he cowrote with physician Frederic J. Mouat, and his own *Charitable and Parochial Establishments* (1881).[19] Architectural historian Jeremy Taylor has described the latter, in fact, as "the first modern textbook on a health care theme by a practising architect."[20] According to his 1904 obituary, Snell was at the time of death one of the two oldest members of the Architectural Association, having joined in 1850. In 1871 or 1873, he became a fellow of the Royal Institute of British Architects.[21]

For Snell and other Victorian architects, architectural practice and even hospital specialization were family affairs. His two sons, Harry Saxon Snell (died 1886) and Alfred Walter Saxon Snell (1860–1949), practiced with him. Alfred Snell carried on his father's legacy, also becoming a leading hospital specialist.[22]

Snell's expertise was determined to a great extent by his early office experience. As a young man, he had worked in the firm of James Pennethorne and acted as assistant to Sir Joseph Paxton, best known as the architect of the Crystal Palace of 1851, and to Sir William Tite. About 1866, he began to work on large public institutions, becoming architect to the St. Marylebone Board of Guardians and building their temporary casual wards. This led to many related commissions. Snell designed an impressive number of workhouses, schools, and infirmaries in England. His unique commitment to hospital design, however, was illustrated by his bequest of £750 at the time of his death for the maintenance of a special triennial scholarship associated with hospital architecture.[23]

The popular reception given Snell's Montreal hospital as a masterpiece may also have been due to its resemblance to two other hospitals, often mentioned by journalists: David Bryce's Royal Infirmary in Edinburgh of 1870 and The Johns Hopkins Hospital in Baltimore, built by John Shaw Billings. Snell knew the Edinburgh building well, as he had visited, drawn, and studied it for his book, *Hospital Construction and Management.* And local legend has it that he had infused the Montreal building with Scottish imagery, such as Scotch thistle decoration in the board room and main corridor, in an attempt to please Smith and Stephen, who had emigrated from Scotland.[24]

The hospital's resemblance to a Scottish castle also linked it to the vernacular traditions established at McGill University. Architects such as Andrew Taylor, who hailed from Edinburgh, designed the university buildings of the 1890s as freestanding limestone pavilions, with raised entries and classical detailing. The pitched copper roofs that transformed to a lovely green with time (and still today provide a dangerous perch for icicles) became a symbol of McGill University, continued in the work of twentieth-century architects such as Percy Nobbs. Indeed, due to the steep ascent of Mount Royal, the view up to the Royal Victoria from Sherbrooke Street across McGill University allows for a strong visual connection between the hospital and campus, especially through the repeating motifs of towers and steep roofs, and the predominance of limestone and copper.

The Pavilion Plan

The basic idea of the pavilion plan was well established by 1893. As Jeremy Taylor has aptly illustrated in *The Architect and the Pavilion Plan,* the type became an international standard in the late nineteenth and early twentieth centuries, with major examples in India, Persia, Russia, Australia, Europe, and North America.[25] The most significant Canadian examples were constructed in the nation's largest cities: the Toronto General Hospital and Montreal's Hôtel-Dieu, the Montreal General Hospital, and the Royal Victoria. First appearing in French hospitals around the time of the French Revolution, and further inspired by the ideas of Florence Nightingale and other midcentury reformers, the concept of separate (or minimally connected) pavilions and the open plan of the wards maximized ventilation in order to discourage miasma, which (it was believed) spread infection.[26] The hallmark of the plan type was the open ward, in which thirty to forty beds were arranged regularly against the outside walls, which in turn were punctuated by a regular rhythm of large windows. The premise was that copious amounts of fresh air circulating between patients would mitigate the chances of contagion.

At first glance, this reliance on fresh air in an 1893 hospital may seem rather old-fashioned. After all, the germ theory of disease transmission had been developed decades earlier, illustrating how "animal and human diseases were caused by distinctive species of microorganisms . . . [that] always came from a previous case of exactly the same disease."[27] While many scholars have suggested that the popularity of the pavilion-plan hospital waned with the development of the germ theory, this was not necessarily so.[28] Public health historian Nancy Tomes has explained how the germ theory did not immediately displace traditional ways of understanding contagion, such as miasma; rather, as the design of the Royal Vic, Johns Hopkins, and many other hospitals illustrates, North Americans incorporated the new theory into traditional explanations (and existing spatial paradigms) for disease.[29] Pavilion-plan hospitals continued to be built into the 1930s.

The Royal Vic as planned and other pavilion-plan hospitals were intended to function as "a great machine" for healing in which fresh air had a crucial function, despite the germ theory.[30] Although the administration block was drastically reduced before construction, a set of drawings by Snell now in the National Archives of Canada gives an overview of his main ideas. As mentioned, the hospital was a modified H-plan, with a five-story central administration block, and rectangular, open wards facing south, with cylindrical towers at their corners. Behind the administration block, both the eastern and western sections of the hospital extended northward, up Mount Royal. To the east this area included the surgical theater and accompanying rooms for professors and students. To the west, along University Street, were a small isolation ward and the medical theater. An extensive pavilion for paying patients and a third ventilating shaft (matching those at the intersections of the ward blocks and administration building) were never built.

The design of the ward itself was a medical instrument by which patients could be carefully positioned in space, according to the gravity of their conditions. As sociologist Lindsay Prior and many hospital architects have noted, the key dimensions of the ward were the distances between beds, the heights of ceilings, and the relationship between windows and beds.[31] Also fundamental to its operation were the relationship between the patients' beds and the nurses' station or desk, and the relationship between the administration building and the pavilion itself.

Early photographs (Figure 1.6) of the Royal Victoria Hospital wards show the general layout of these huge rectangular spaces. White metal beds were arranged along the exterior walls of the long and narrow wards.[32] Most photos show a less-than-ideal arrangement by which more than one bed was positioned between pairs of windows. Even a version of Snell's plan that illustrates the placement of thirty-two beds, published in 1913, shows pairs of beds between each window.[33]

And although the idea was to minimize crowding, the circulation area in the center of the ward, defined by the ends of the beds, was typically strewn with rocking chairs, as well as desks and tables for the use of nurses. The gigantic central radiators, each topped with a marble slab, became makeshift tables.[34] A large round institutional clock hung at the south end of the ward. Nearly every extant photo of the wards, for example, the striking 1912 photo of the Typhoid ward (Figure 1.7), shows the space embellished with plants, perhaps in an effort to soften the room's massive scale and institutional appearance.[35]

An extraordinary fragment of a plan (Figure 1.8), labeled Sick Ward, shows the architect's careful dimensioning of the room and the framing of the floor. The Royal Victoria Hospital wards, according to hospital secretary and superintendent John J. Robson, were 123 feet × 26 feet 6 inches and 14 feet high.[36] Snell was an expert on the issue of ward size, having published a lengthy explanation of the relationship of ward size to other costs in 1888. In this same article, Snell described the ideal ward as accommodating between twenty and thirty-two patients.[37] In *Charitable and Parochial Establishments,* he had recommended a combination of casement and lifting sash windows, to prevent drafts on patients in bed (Figure 1.9), a combination the architect had previously used at

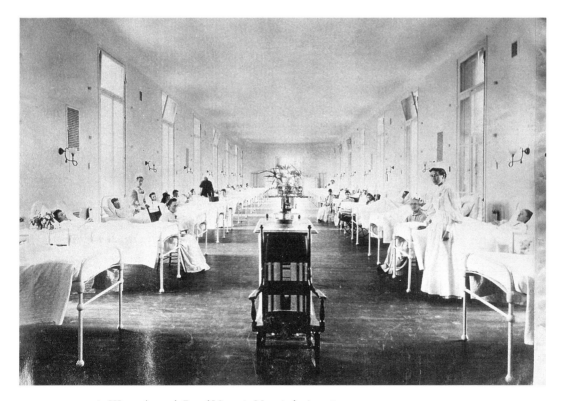

FIGURE 1.6. Women's ward, Royal Victoria Hospital, circa 1894.

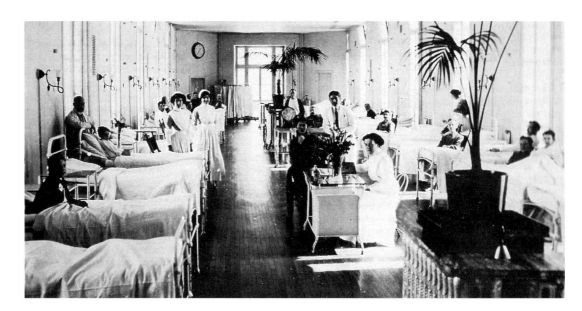

FIGURE 1.7. Typhoid ward, Royal Victoria Hospital.

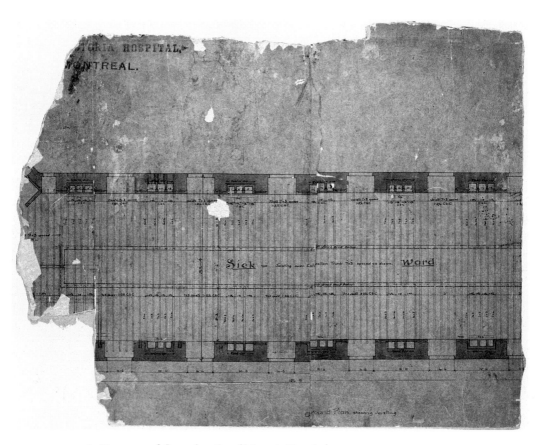

FIGURE 1.8. Fragment of floor plan, Royal Victoria Hospital.

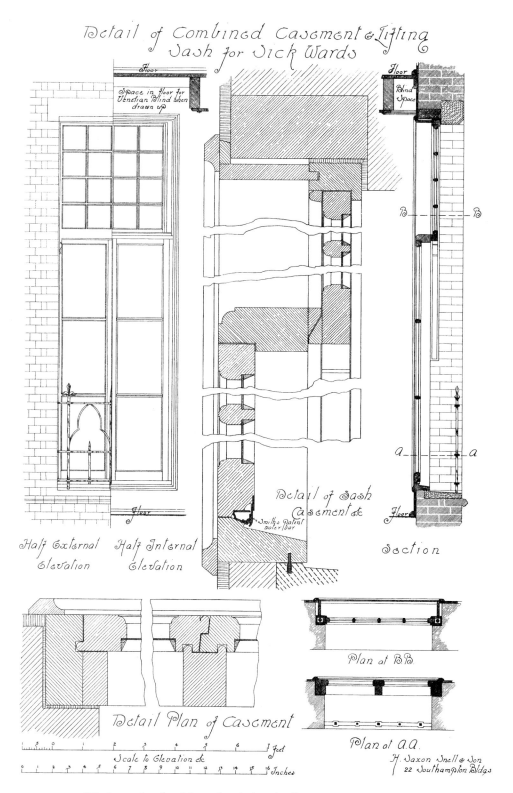

Detail of Combined Casement & Lifting
Sash for Sick Wards

Floor

Space in floor for
Venetian Blind when
drawn up

Floor

Blind
Space

B ———— B

a ———— a

Floor

Detail of Sash
Casement &c

Smith's Patent
roller bar

Section

Half External
Elevation

Half Internal
Elevation

Detail Plan of Casement

Plan at BB.

Plan at a.a.

Scale to Elevation &c

1 Feet

Inches

H. Saxon Snell & Son
22 Southampton Bldgs

FIGURE 1.9. Window sashes for sick wards, window detail.

St. George's Union, St. Olave's, and Holborn Union infirmaries. A full-scale drawing in the John Bland Canadian Architecture Collection illustrates how Snell's windows at the Royal Victoria Hospital operated. A photograph (Figure 1.6) shows the ward's casement windows open, flushing the expansive room with fresh air.

Another important attribute of the open ward was that a single nurse could supervise a large group of patients. Nightingale, whose name is often linked with wards and pavilion-plan design, believed that the close surveillance of patients by nurses was essential to modern care. "The design of an ideal hospital for Nightingale was bound up with notions of cleanliness, order, observation and education," explains architectural historian Cynthia Hammond.[38] Nightingale criticized Snell's plan for the Royal Vic, especially its lost opportunities for ward supervision. "Duty room is as far from the Ward as it can be," she wrote in January 1888. "In fact should be called off-duty room."[39]

Images such as the photo of typhoid patients in a Royal Victoria Hospital ward in 1912 (Figure 1.7) show a nurse sitting at a white table or desk, facing one long wall, located about halfway down the long space. Proximity to the patients and the openness of the plan allowed nurses to respond instantly to patients' needs. Interestingly, the same arrangement of a supervisory work station overlooking a group of potentially disorderly users would become popular nearly a half century later in middle-class domestic architecture and other female work spaces, such as schools and libraries.[40] Post–World War II houses, which typically featured a kitchen open to a multipurpose room, permitted mothers to cook, clean, and watch children from a single position.[41]

The wards of the Royal Victoria Hospital, and many other hospitals constructed in the late nineteenth century, were laid out according to the so-called group system, whereby medical and surgical (and sometimes special as well) patients were accommodated in separate quarters. European hospitals were well known for this arrangement; in England, the hospitals at Manchester and Glasgow Royal Infirmary were "some excellent examples of this grouping."[42] In addition to the distinctive wards of the pavilion-plan hospital, at least four other spatial features were fundamental to the operation of the hospital in 1893: operating theaters, the system of ventilation, arrangements for isolation, and staff quarters.

Operating Theaters

The surgical amphitheater, most medical historians suggest, was a direct descendant of the much older anatomical theater.[43] Early-nineteenth-century surgical amphitheaters, like those in New York and Philadelphia, were typically rather grand circular or semicircular spaces with steeply tiered seating. In these theaters, the surgeon would perform the operation on a patient, who was lying on a bed or stretcher on a stagelike area illuminated by a skylight. And although their primary function was to instruct doctors-to-be in the methods of surgery, these public operations also served as a form of rather grisly public entertainment, as anatomical demonstrations had served in previous centuries.

An additional reason for having an entirely separate space for the provision of surgery, as this passage from 1845 concerning the Pennsylvania Hospital makes clear, was to protect other patients from the sights and sounds of surgery. Acoustic insulation became increasingly significant with the growing number of accidents resulting from urban industrialization:

The want of a room on the same floor as the Surgical ward in which operations may be done and the patients afterwards kept until their more dangerous Symptoms have subsided, has been long apparent, and at the present time in consequence of the increase of serious accidents is particularly felt. The subjects brought into the house with bad fractures from railroads, machinery &c are generally upon arrival at the Hospital in a state of exhaustion and are brought into a condition to undergo an operation only by the administration of stimuli, and are liable to serious losses of blood upon the slightest motion—in such patients removal from the bed and rooms in which they may be first placed to the present operating theatre is always painful and dangerous and in many instances is utterly impracticable, and no ward being at present devoted to this purpose, the painful mutilations which such accidents often demand must consequently be done in the presence of the other patients. The bad effects resulting to men in many instances but a few degrees better off than the actual sufferer from the sight of bloody operations and the cries and complaints of the patient, it is needless to dwell upon. Your Medical Officers strenuously urge in any contemplated improvements, that a room be fitted up in an appropriate manner for the reception of such accidents as are likely to require operative aid, and such as from the severity of their injuries are likely to survive but for a short period. They would suggest for this purpose the North room of the East wing on the lower floor.[44]

The opportunities for drama in the surgical theater were well known to surgeons. The period following the introduction of anesthesia (1840s) and the acceptance of prophylactic surgical antisepsis "marked the summit of the surgeon's dazzling actor-role, in which the spotlight of the public gaze was focused upon him."[45] In major metropolitan areas, such as London, hundreds of people might attend operations (only a handful would become surgeons), and the end of the surgical procedure was often marked by thunderous applause.

This "performance" by surgeons was thus markedly different from that of nurses. Surgeons controlled the timing of their shows and performed for a discerning audience increasingly made up of men who wanted to emulate them, in a setting that consciously reminded viewers of their position as audience members, keeping them, literally, in their place. In this way, "onstage" and "backstage" were separate for surgeons. By contrast, nurses were on view all the time, for an audience of poor people who didn't necessarily aspire to become nurses, in a setting that naturalized the mutual gaze between nurse and patient, while offering no boundaries whatsoever between their spaces. Indeed, nurses moved among and between patients in order to do their jobs. What's more, when nurses were housed in the ward, "onstage" and "backstage" were completely merged.[46]

By 1893, the surgical amphitheater in new hospitals was typically a smaller-scaled, elegantly designed space, intended only for the instruction of medical students and physicians.[47] Its special location and careful design are evidence of the growing acceptance of surgery as a major medical intervention, and the increasing prestige of surgery as a specialty among physicians. The design of so-called surgical suites, the type that succeeded the theater in the teaching hospital, is commonly listed among the reasons that middle-class patients opted to use the institution in the 1920s.[48] The design of such surgical suites, an arrangement of smaller rooms usually occupying the end of a double-loaded corridor, is discussed in chapter 5.

Notman's photographs (Figures 1.10 and 1.11) of two theaters at the Royal Vic show the interim state of this transformation from public theater to private suite. These

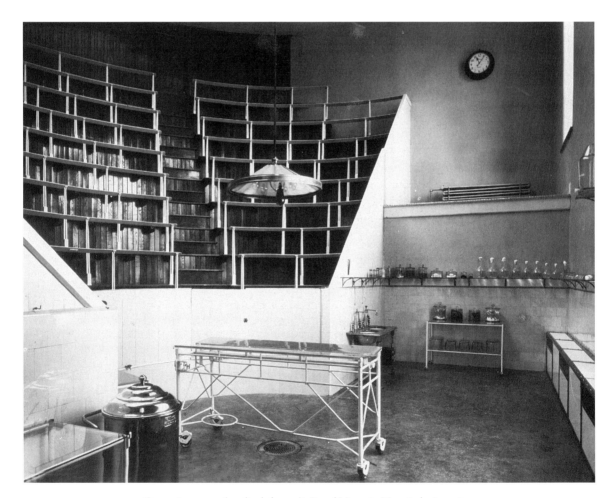

FIGURE 1.10. Operating room (medical theater), Royal Victoria Hospital, circa 1894.

theaters were located directly behind and above the open wards, north of the ventilating towers (at the top of the H), on the east and west sides of the hospital. Both theaters appear flooded in natural light; taken from one end of the "performance" space, the photos reveal the proximity of students and their instructors at this time, even though Notman photographed them empty. Compared to a famous photograph (Figure 1.12) of a dissection, taken in 1884, the new space designed for teaching less than a decade later appears airy, orderly, clean, rational, and modern.

Snell produced detailed drawings for both the medical and the surgical theaters, illustrating the importance of the spaces in the building program. Both theaters were rectangular structures, with steep gabled roofs, connected to the hospital by a narrower corridor. The main level comprised semicircular, tiered seating, positioned to allow visitors views of procedures that took place along the long elevation of the building. The medical theater purportedly sat 200 or 250 students, and adjoined professors' private rooms

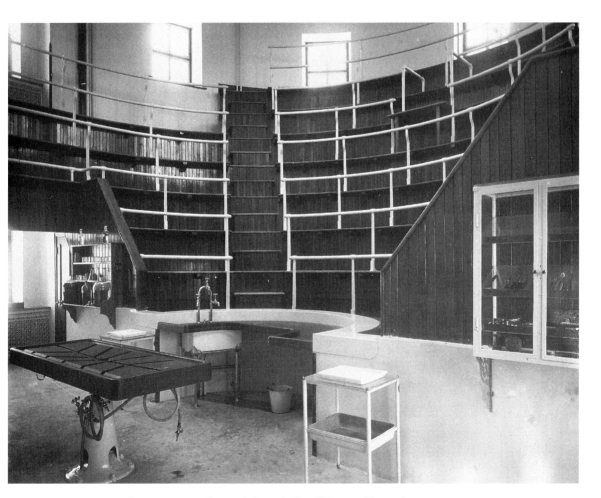

FIGURE 1.11. Operating room (surgical theater), Royal Victoria Hospital, circa 1894.

and the patients' waiting room on the ground floor of the staircase block.[49] The space below the seating is labeled "students room." Above, the main theater was illuminated by two large windows set into the roof, and two smaller skylights along the ridgeline. Behind the instructor were four tall, narrow windows. The north end of the building appears in an image (Figure 1.13) probably intended to document the pathology wing added to the building subsequent to its opening.

Snell's surgical theater (Figure 1.14), too, as drawn in February 1892, was roughly fifty-three feet by forty-four feet, and was minimally connected to its (west) ward tower, and to support rooms for anesthesia and instruments, by a small corridor (level with the floor of the theater) with four windows. On the ground floor, beneath the theater seats, was a room for students' "hats & cloaks" and an adjacent washroom (eight urinals, two toilets).[50] Medical students were intended to enter the theater directly from the exterior (northeast corner), through a small lobby, and then to take iron stairways located along the back wall to their special seating.

Snell drew floor plans at both ten feet and five feet to the inch. The larger-scale (undated) plan (Figure 1.15), a remarkable drawing that shows both levels of the theater simultaneously, is accompanied by a splendid detail of the students' seats. The distance between the cast-iron standards that differentiated each level of seat was two feet; each standard was three feet high. The rhythm of change—seat, step, seat—was paced at one foot, an indication of how carefully the space was designed for student observers, rather than for the patient.

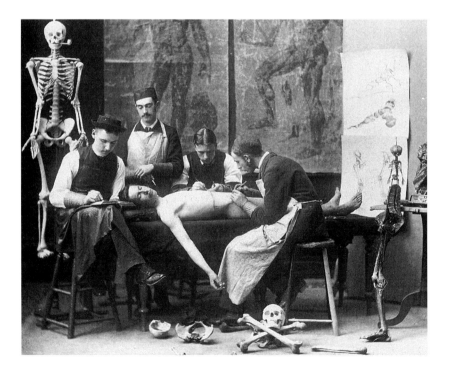

FIGURE 1.12.
Anatomy study,
McGill medical
students, Montreal,
1884.

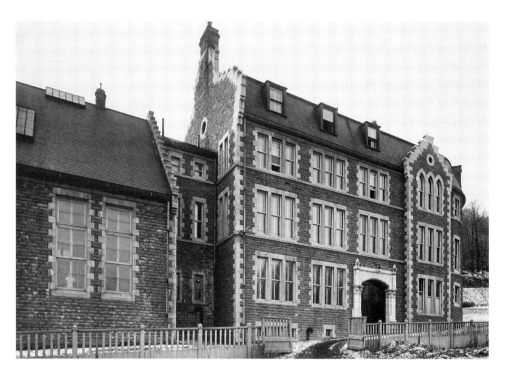

FIGURE 1.13. Pathology Building, Royal Victoria Hospital, circa 1894.

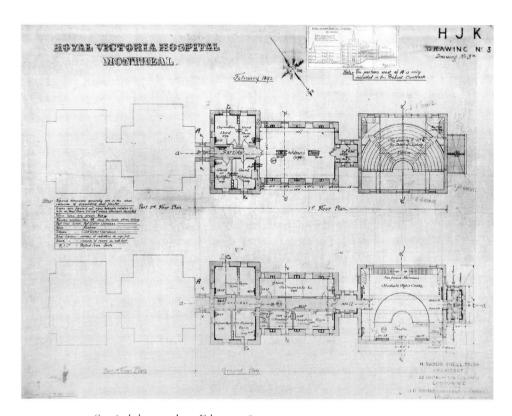

FIGURE 1.14. Surgical theater plans, February 1892.

The most complex architectural feature of the surgical and medical theaters at the Royal Vic was the design to maximize natural illumination. Just over twenty-four feet above the theater floor, a glass gable popped up from the main section of the slate roof and presumably flooded the space with natural light, augmented by a huge window in the northeast wall, behind the surgeon. A series of hinged panels (called "ceiling lights" in the drawing) made it possible to close off the lantern, too.

A large-scale (five feet = one inch) section (Figure 1.16) by Snell shows both the framing of this generous lantern and its elevation. Small windows ring the entire lantern (eight on the long side; five on the short side), just below the copper roof. Two small ventilators also punctuated Snell's roof. The architect noted on the drawings that the ventilators on the surgical and medical theaters were similar.

Notably absent from the Snell-designed theaters are the support rooms, such as the series constructed at contemporary theaters, both the Fenwick Operating Theater at the Kingston General Hospital (1894), in Kingston, Ontario, and the Pemberton Operating Theater (1896; additions 1918) at the Royal Jubilee Hospital in Victoria, British Columbia, to meet the complex requirements of surgery. These two examples, both extant today,

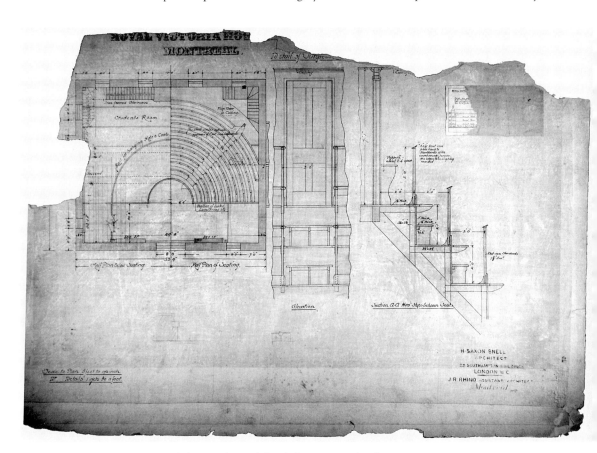

FIGURE 1.15. Surgical theater plan and detailed section, undated.

show the variations in operating theater design at the time of the Royal Victoria Hospital. The Kingston hospital included rooms for doctors to change, wash, and consult before the surgeries, and a separate preparatory room for anesthetizing patients. The original Pemberton theater included one sterilizing room; a second one was added in 1918. Perhaps most significantly, though, two postoperative recovery rooms were added to the wooden corridor that linked the operating theater to the main hospital. Perhaps at the Royal Victoria some of these ancillary procedures took place in the theater itself, since the photographs show the presence of equipment. Other furnishings in the amphitheater were of "great use and practicability": an iron screen for displaying diagrams, an iron stool for the examination of patients, and an apparatus for projections.[51]

Student spectators were fundamental to the ways these surgical theaters functioned. Both Royal Victoria Hospital theaters and the Fenwick, as previously mentioned, included tiered seating for spectators. This was typical in large teaching hospitals at this time across North America. The Pemberton (Figure 1.17), on the other hand, was a much more modest space, accommodating only the surgical staff and patient. It follows the earlier penchant for separation from the general hospital per se, while foreshadowing the

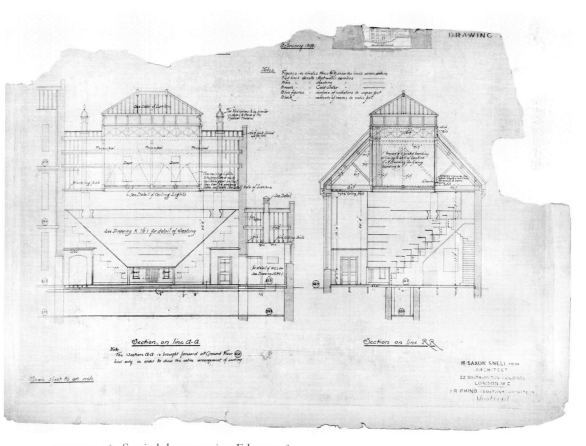

FIGURE 1.16. Surgical theater section, February 1892.

less theatrical (and considerably more intimate) requirements of the post–World War I surgeon (as we will see in chapter 5).

The Pemberton operating room's unique design follows closely Joseph Lister's principles of antiseptic surgery as they were embraced in Canada. The techniques of antiseptic surgery, which consisted of using carbolic acid as an antiseptic spray and sound dressing in order to reduce the risk of postoperative infections, had been studied by Royal Jubilee surgeon J. C. Davie while he was in Europe on sabbatical.[52] The premium placed on light, air, and easy-to-clean materials (notably mosaic tile and plastered walls) by the architect of the Pemberton operating room also illustrates the full acceptance, by this time, of the germ theory; its adjacent sterilizing rooms are evidence of the relatively new custom of sterilizing surgical instruments. It is tempting to speculate, too, that the reduced scale of the Victoria theater might have been in an effort to neutralize the air's infective properties (following Louis Pasteur's ideas in the 1860s) and to decrease exposure of the patient.

Ventilation

The need for proper ventilation permeated nearly every scale of the pavilion-plan hospital, from its site design to the architect's choice of window hardware. We have already

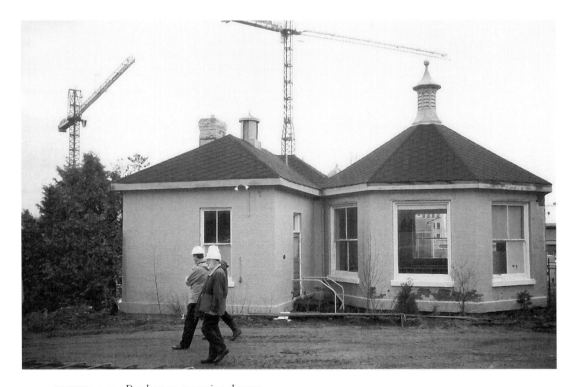

FIGURE 1.17. Pemberton operating theater.

looked briefly at the architecture of open wards, which were designed to surround patients in natural light and fresh air. Snell was very concerned about fresh air. Debates raged among his British architectural colleagues in the 1890s about the proper way to ventilate pavilion-plan hospitals. While the arrangement of the pavilion-plan hospital itself encouraged passive cross-ventilation, some architects experimented with mechanical means, too. William Henman, for example, completely retrofitted his design for the 346-bed Birmingham hospital in 1892–93. On December 7, 1893 (a mere five days after the opening of the Montreal building), Henman patented the design of a purifying screen, placed at the head of each bed, presumably to clean the air.[53] Following his letter written to the *Builder* in 1896, Henman secured the commission for the Royal Victoria Hospital in Belfast (1900–1903), which according to Taylor forever changed the direction of hospital architecture.[54] Instead of separate pavilions, the Belfast hospital featured seventeen top-lit, windowless wards arranged contiguously along a single connecting corridor. This new arrangement was possible because the hospital was ventilated mechanically, foreshadowing Le Corbusier's unbuilt windowless hospital proposed for Venice in 1965.

Snell's precise position in the great debate over natural versus mechanical ventilation favored the former. This is clearly articulated both in his texts and his architecture. By 1913, Alfred Saxon Snell remained unconvinced of the Belfast system: "The Belfast type is unique and likely to remain so. It was designed to fit a system of mechanical ventilation which has—I venture to think fortunately—failed, so far, to secure general approval for use in connection with hospitals."[55] The younger Snell was also an advocate of single- rather than multistory pavilions. As these were not common in England, he pointed to hospitals in both Germany and France as models: the Berlin Virchow Hospital (opened in 1906) and the Rothschild Hospital, "now nearing completion in Paris."[56]

In terms of the actual air space provided per bed at the Royal Victoria Hospital, Snell's position was fairly moderate. As he pointed out in 1888, other hospital experts recommended anywhere from 1,200 to 2,000 cubic feet per patient; a committee appointed to consider the same question concluded that 850 cubic feet was a minimum for each hospital patient. Four hospitals Snell had designed prior to 1888, he boasted, provided 950 cubic feet per person.[57] And the wards at the Royal Vic were, at 123 feet by 26 feet 6 inches, only slightly larger than his suggested ideal size of 120 feet long and 24 feet wide.[58]

The heating and ventilating of Montreal's Royal Victoria are an interesting chapter in these ongoing debates over natural versus mechanical ventilation systems in pavilion-plan institutions. Dr. John Shaw Billings, who designed and oversaw the construction of the influential Johns Hopkins Hospital, had suggested that fireplaces "waste fuel, increase labor, cause noise and dust, and are somewhat dangerous," in addition to heating hospitals insufficiently (as the outside temperature approaches freezing). But Snell defended the use of fireplaces for heating: "The opinions here expressed as to the utility and value of open fireplaces in large sick wards is [sic] not shared by those in this country who have made the subject their special study."[59]

Snell's original scheme of 1889 apparently called for sixty fireplaces to heat the administration building. These may have been the Thermhydric fireplaces he had patented and specified in at least four of his British buildings.[60] On a set of drawings for the administration building dated December 1889, however, these fireplaces are not shown.[61]

The Royal Victoria Hospital board found Snell's heating plan inadequate. J. W. Hopkins, a local architect, government architect Thomas Fuller, and heating contractor Charles Garth looked at Snell's drawings and "gave an unfavourable report."[62] According to a memorandum by the hospital, Hopkins drew up alternative heating plans. Snell then traveled to Montreal and attended a meeting on May 3, 1889. He disapproved of the suggested changes to the heating of the building and declared that he would not be responsible for ensuing problems. Revised plans arrived in January 1890, incorporating a system of central heating. According to hospital historian David Sclater Lewis, it was decided to retain the chimneys from the original scheme, even though the fireplaces had been omitted in the revised plans.[63] Today these chimneys are still visible in the building's silhouette.

Snell and John Abbott had exchanged words on the benefits of steam and hot water heating; Snell apparently favored steam, while Abbott pointed to other Montreal buildings. "Steam heating has for sometime been almost entirely abandoned in the City, and hot water heating is practically universal," he wrote in a letter to the architect dated March 26, 1889.[64] The final building incorporated a system of hot water heating, with separate furnaces in the basement of each building; shortly after 1900 this system was again changed.

Contemporary descriptions of the hospital suggest that fresh air entered the wards through gratings in the ceilings; warm air entered through a small square inlet (Figure 1.18). This cold air was then heated to about eighty degrees by passing over steam coils. Foul air, on the other hand, was removed through two series of gratings, one near the floor and one at a height of six feet from the floor. Ducts from these led to the large flue in the center of each wing. In warm weather, of course, the floor-to-ceiling windows served to further ventilate the wards.[65] Snell's drawings also specify Tobin's tubes and Arnott's ventilators, popular Victorian devices especially designed to ventilate interior spaces, in the walls beside the fireplaces.[66]

Snell's detailed drawings of the towers (Figure 1.19), like his plans for the theaters, are impressive. They show how the architect's strategy for ventilation shaped the general massing of the building. Robson claimed that the large ventilating shaft in the center of the tower drew the foul air from all the adjoining wards. In the center of the chimney rose the smoke shaft from the boilers in the basement, which "materially assists the draught power."[67] Unfortunately, Snell said little about how these towers were supposed to work. In a brief quote in the *Canadian Architect and Builder* of 1889, he outlined the way the vertical organization of the building section, particularly the lack of stairs, was intended to prevent the spread of foul air:

I have had more difficulty in designing the plan for this hospital than any other I built. This is accounted for by the peculiarity of the Canadian climate, its intense heat and cold. For instance, hospital buildings in the south of France would in nowise do here. There they are built upon the hut plan, and of course that is the proper plan for all hospitals. But were that plan followed here, it would cost a fortune every winter for fuel alone; for in that system the hospital is scattered over a large tract of land and is only one storey high, and consists of a number of separate buildings. So it will be seen how difficult it would be to build such a hospital as that in Montreal, as each building has to have a separate heating apparatus. It is always difficult to prevent foul air from reaching the upper storeys in hospitals not built on the hut plan, as it always travels by the stairway. I have taken means in my plan of the present hospital to prevent this, by detaching the stair case, and putting on each floor short bridges, so that there will be no staircase for it to ascend.[68]

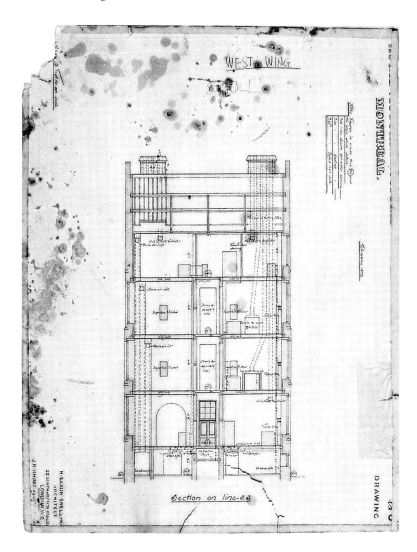

FIGURE 1.18.
Section showing
ventilation, Royal
Victoria Hospital.

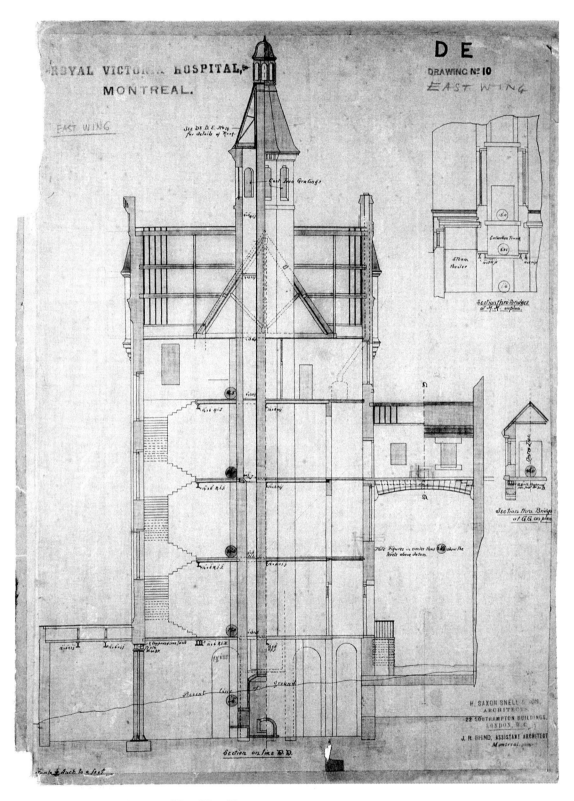

FIGURE 1.19. Section of East Wing Tower.

British hospital architects were particularly proud of their design of sanitary facilities, and quick to compare their own standards to those of both Europe and the United States. The main difference was that toilets in British hospitals were frequently accommodated in disconnected and thus heavily ventilated spaces, like the towers at the Royal Vic. Typical examples are the towers at King's College Hospital, by William Pite, and Edwin Hall's Manchester Royal Infirmary. And the pattern endured, even long after architects like Alfred Saxon Snell considered the separation irrelevant. He designed an ideal pavilion in 1912 with a disconnected sanitary tower. To avoid blocking the southern exposure, however, Snell's ideal tower was located to the east of the ward (Figure 1.20). Thus Johns Hopkins, "one of the best hospitals in the United States, and one of the most celebrated pavilion hospitals in the world," was considered inferior to British hospitals in terms of sanitary facilities.[69] "Even the new model Hospital at Baltimore, the result of an examination of the best modern hospitals of Europe, is far from perfect in this respect," reported the *Builder* in 1884.[70]

ISOLATION

Not unrelated to the issue of ventilation was the isolation of patients. Snell's plan for the Royal Vic included special rooms for particularly contagious patients. In 1888, he advised that rooms for such patients should be "attached to the large ward, but not so as to communicate with it directly," exactly as he designed for the Montreal hospital.[71] The plan as published in the *Builder* shows these smaller "separation wards" at the north ends of the surgical and medical wards. They appear as rather nondescript square rooms, not unlike the rooms for nurses and medical officers and the ward kitchen, with which

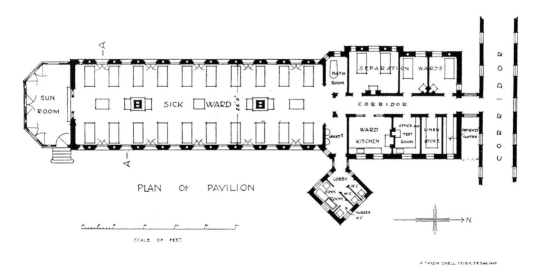

FIGURE 1.20. A. Saxon Snell, ideal, disconnected sanitary tower.

they were grouped. Just north of the ventilating tower, too, was a block of separation wards planned by Snell. In a detailed description of the building written in 1894, private and isolation wards are also said to be on the fourth story of the medical wing, "so arranged that the nurse in charge can have no need of communication with either the private or public wards."[72] Indeed, Snell's interior elevations show rectangular windows (see Figure 1.18), designed to observe patients from an adjacent space, termed "inspection windows."

In the architect's mind, however, most infectious cases would go to a separate infectious hospital located on the same site: four smaller, rectangular buildings planned for a distance of four hundred feet behind the mortuary. It was included in a plan (Figure 1.21) published in the *Builder* as late as July 1893. Snell was asked to cut costs midway through the process, however, and the final building omitted both this isolation hospital and his planned outpatients' department.[73] The administration building, too, was reduced considerably in 1890. The differences between the architect's intentions in 1889, and what was eventually built, are evident by comparing two sets of drawings now in the John Bland Canadian Architecture Collection. Five undated plans (scale one-tenth to an inch) show in remarkable detail Snell's ideal administration building, including room names, dimensions, and framing. Two drawings even retain the brass tacks presumably used to suspend alternative ideas, perhaps during meetings. A second undated set shows a considerably smaller building. These plans for a reduced building are signed off on by the hospital's administration.

Like a miniaturized model of the pavilion-plan hospital (although oriented to the east), Snell's never-built infectious hospital had a central administration building for staff and separate pavilions for the patients. In this case, however, the pavilions had no connection to the central building and were lifted off the ground, sitting on an "open" basement. Two of the buildings had two, six-bed wards, kitchen, and sanitary facilities; the other two contained four-bed wards, also with kitchens, sanitary facilities, and a private patient's room. Deluxe indeed was this room for an infectious patient, with three exterior walls. These details may seem trivial now, since Snell's infectious hospital was never built; they do provide insight, nonetheless, into current thinking about the (ideal) isolation of patients in 1893. Certain details, too (such as the highly exposed room), show how the seeds of subsequent architectural developments were sown even before the twentieth century began.

This foreshadowing of later issues in hospital building is particularly true regarding tensions between clients and architects. What was the value of Snell's expertise? A bitter dispute arose over the architect's 5 percent fee, which Snell thought should be based on the larger, unbuilt scheme.[74] Abbott, writing to Royal Vic benefactor George Stephen in February 1891 about the architect's estimate of building costs, noted the considerable difference between the version of the building in the architect's imagination and that depicted in the plans:

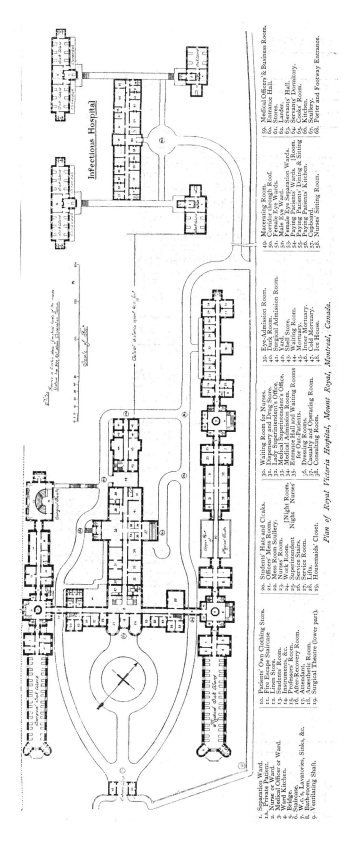

Infectious Hospital

1. Separation Ward.
1A. Private Patient.
2. Nurse or Ward.
3. Medical Officer or Ward.
4. Ward Kitchen.
5. Bridge.
6. Staircase.
7. W.c.'s, Lavatories, Sinks, &c.
8. Bath-room.
9. Ventilating Shaft.

10. Patients' Own Clothing Store.
11. Fire Escape Staircase.
12. Linen Store.
13. Students' Room.
14. Instruments, &c.
15. Professors' Room.
16. After-Recovery Room.
17. Attendant.
18. Anaesthetic Room.
19. Surgical Theatre (lower part).

20. Students' Hats and Cloaks.
21. Officers' Mess Room.
22. Mess Room Scullery.
23. Nurses' Room.
24. Work Room.   [Night Room.
25. Superintendent   Night Nurses'
26. Service Stairs.
27. Service Room.
28. Lifts.
29. Housemaids' Closet.

30. Waiting Room for Nurses.
31. Dispensary and Drug Store.
32. Lady Superintendent's Office.
33. Medical Superintendent's Office.
34. Medical Admission Room.
35. Entrance Hall and Waiting Rooms
        for Out-Patients.
36. Dressing Rooms.
37. Casualty and Operating Room.
38. Consulting Room.

39. Eye-Admission Room.
40. Dark Room.
41. Surgical Admission Room.
42. Yard.
43. Shell Store.
44. Waiting Room.
45. Mortuary.
46. Inner Mortuary.
47. Cold Mortuary.
48. Ice House.

49. Macerating Room.
50. Corridor through Roof.
51. Female Eye Wards.
52. Male Eye Ward.
53. Female Eye Separation Wards.
54. Paying Patients' Wards. [Room.
55. Paying Patients' Dining & Sitting
56. Paying Patients' Kitchen.
57. Cupboard.
58. Nurses' Sitting Room.

59. Medical Officers' & Business Room.
60. Entrance Hall.
61. Stores.
62. Larder.
63. Servants' Hall.
64. Servants' Dormitory.
65. Cooks' Room.
66. Kitchen.
67. Scullery.
68. Porter and Footway Entrance.

Plan of Royal Victoria Hospital, Mount Royal, Montreal, Canada.

FIGURE 1.21. Original plan of the Royal Victoria Hospital.

I am sorry to have so bad an account to give you of Mr. Snell. . . . [The estimate] applied to the whole building as he has had it in his head and not to the plans with which has furnished us. . . . [He] really seems to have no common sense at all, however good a designer of hospitals he may be.[75]

A series of terse letters passed between Abbott and Snell in 1891, mostly dealing with their varying recollections of the agreements between the hospital board and the architect. This negative account of Snell on the part of the hospital president is ironic in retrospect, given that much of the building's early acclaim, at least in the press, came from the board's choice of architect.

Staff Quarters

The residences and offices for staff in the original architecture of the Royal Victoria Hospital were scattered all over the complex. The administration building, not surprisingly, had the highest density of staff offices. The ground floor included the offices of the board, the secretary (and staff), and the steward (and staff). Resident medical officers, according to the description in the *Montreal Medical Journal*, were also "quartered" here.

On Snell's plans, the first floor, as it was called, was fully occupied by nurses. Rooms along the facade included the bedroom for the Lady Superintendent; directly over the entrance was the library for nurses, with a dining room (west) and sitting room for nurses on either side. Most of the second floor and at least some of the third (the plan is torn), too, were dedicated to nurses. Medical officers slept on the ground floor, to the east of the main entry. The fourth floor contained the kitchen and scullery in the central section, with maids and housekeepers to the east (by this height the east is already roof). The fifth (top) floor, occupied only in the central section, included ten maids' rooms off a central, double-loaded corridor.

Why so many hospital employees needed to live in the hospital is a question never answered directly in the primary sources. Perhaps the opportunity to live in the palatial structure on the slopes of Mount Royal, surrounded by the extensive and well-maintained grounds, was a way to attract good staff. On September 2, 1897, a number of medical luminaries enjoyed a garden party on the "beautiful grounds of the Royal Victoria Hospital" as part of the British Medical Association's first meeting outside of Britain. Newspaper accounts of the social function pointed to the hospital's paradoxical image of an up-to-date medical facility contained within a picturesque castle, like the cultural historian Leo Marx's celebrated metaphor of machine in the garden: "It looked yesterday more like some English place which had taken ages for the perfection of its exquisite lawns and terraces than the result of a few short years. It shows what care and cultivation can do. . . . The pathological and bacteriological laboratories held much interest for the profession. They are so fully equipped—'perfect' is again the only word—in every detail."[76]

CONCLUSION

Traditional and high-tech, modern yet comforting, the central issues of twentieth-century hospital design were suggested before 1900. Our close encounter with the Royal Victoria Hospital and its sources leading up to and on its opening day has shown how a hospital functioned in a variety of urban roles, ranging from a tourist monument to a castle for the sick poor and a comfortable home for health-care workers. Debates about location, charity, and technical expertise meant that design intentions were compromised in the name of progress.

The resulting Royal Victoria Hospital as a case study illustrates the careful balance sought after by architects and administrators. A new hospital had to look like others—indeed, the RVH was instantly recognizable as a pavilion-plan building—yet also seem distinctive and regionally inspired. Extant drawings by the Snell firm show how the open ward, its furniture, and surgical theaters were designed to function as complex healing technologies. The larger hospital, too, was arranged to maximize air and light and sometimes facilitate patient isolation, in ways that did not always correspond with medical thinking of 1893. These issues, especially expertise, patronage, domesticity, and modernization, will become the subjects of intense discussion in the ensuing decades, particularly among design and health-care professionals. As in 1893, these debates are legible in the built environment.

Patients

2 IN ONE OF A SERIES OF ARTICLES ANTICIPATING THE AMERICAN HOS-
pital Association conference in Montreal in October 1920, the influential Chicago-based journal *Modern Hospital* described the four-year-old
Ross Memorial Pavilion at Montreal's Royal Victoria Hospital as "the
final word of the day in hospital construction and architecture."[1] Photographs of the hospital (Figure 2.1) taken from a distance show how
Boston-based architects Stevens and Lee, North America's most prominent hospital architects, sited the Ross Memorial Pavilion to appear as
a kind of crown to the older hospital. Located just behind and above
the pavilion-plan building, as the photograph shows, it blurred the picturesque, serrated outline of Snell's sprawling complex by obscuring
its irregular rooflines and chimneys. Just as the city's most luxurious
houses towered over others in Montreal, the new private patients' pavilion communicated the powerful economic status of its users: "It naturally dominates the group when viewed from a distance," reported an
observant journalist.[2]

Just what was so fashionable about the Ross? Perhaps the journalist
was referring to its standing as a private patients' pavilion. Unlike those
who frequented Snell's pavilion-plan hospital, patients at the Ross were
mostly wealthy Montrealers, who, when sick, chose to separate themselves from the general public in luxurious quarters. Indeed, by 1918,

private rooms and surgical suites fulfilled the functions formerly satisfied by the open wards, separate isolation hospitals, and surgical theaters of the pavilion-plan buildings that had preceded them.

This chapter looks at the accommodation of four new groups of patients in hospitals of the 1920s and 1930s using the same methodology as chapter 1, juxtaposing architectural drawings, extant hospitals, and other primary sources. Paying patients, outpatients, pregnant women, and children inspired new spatial challenges. Some of these were controlled by regulations, while others were met through architectural solutions. The argument, taken up again in chapter 4, is that planning overtook ventilation as the major concern of hospital architects about the time of World War I. The Ross Pavilion and the handful of institutions for paying patients built after the end of World War I were not simply expansions in the physical plant of older hospitals but rather were examples of a new type of hospital building.

The period from 1880 to 1939 saw hospitals undergo sharp social divisions. Many hospitals or parts of hospitals continued to function socially as a form of charitable assistance to the poor, as we saw in chapter 1. But in addition to this continuing responsibility, many hospitals took on new obligations. New hospitals anticipated and responded to a number of contrasting special interests: municipal versus private, religious

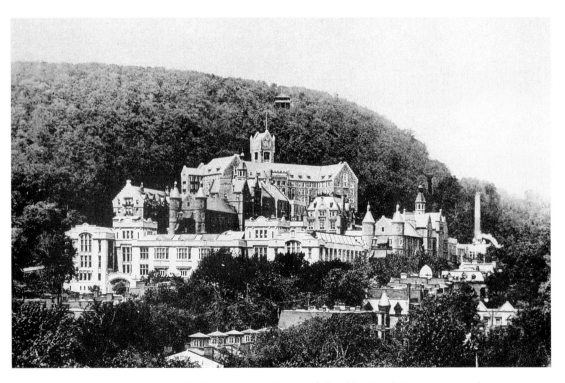

FIGURE 2.1. Ross Memorial Pavilion crowned the site of the older Royal Victoria Hospital, reflecting its economic function to attract paying patients.

versus lay, Catholic versus Protestant, convalescent versus acute, women versus men, French versus English, and rich patients versus poor ones. These divisions were especially visible in Montreal, where linguistic and religious differences had long controlled education, health care, and other social services.

As historians of medicine have noted, hospitals retained the general intention to care for the poor, but the overall goal of the hospital system became to cure the sick. The procedures, equipment, and architecture required to cure people differed from those required to care for the poor. Thus, although there was stimulation for hospital development in changing medical procedures, the problem of finding suitable ways of attracting and accommodating a broadened clientele—all of society—stimulated architectural activity, too.

To entice new patients, hospitals developed a nuanced set of responses to different people based on a combination of medical theory and social analysis. In the case of the poor patient, the hospital experience was intended to differ from home life: reduced responsibilities, better food, and cleaner, quieter, and more restful surroundings. We saw in chapter 1 how Snell's castlelike design projected images of a decidedly Scottish and vaguely European aristocratic past on poor Montrealers. For the middle-class patient, however, the post–World War I hospital had to duplicate or even surpass the standards established in the domestic environment he or she knew at home. This domestic ideology is evident in buildings like the Ross Pavilion and differs from the "big house" image we will see in the development of the nurses' residence in chapter 3. For while domestic imagery in the nurses' residence smoothed the transition for middle-class women to the world of work outside the home, homey ideology in private patients' pavilions was intended to attract much-needed financial support for the expanding institution by signaling hospitality. As a precedent for new hospitals, then, the European castle was surpassed by the modern hotel.

Paying Patients

The phenomenon of purpose-built pavilions for private patients was widespread but short-lived. Following the stock market crash of 1929, the demand for costly accommodation dropped off considerably, and many private patients' pavilions were refurbished for alternative uses. The case of the Montreal General Hospital (MGH) is a typical reuse scenario. As early as 1890, doctors were lured from the Montreal General Hospital to the Royal Victoria because of its superior accommodation for paying patients. In 1930, the Montreal General Hospital constructed a private patients' pavilion on the site of the Western Hospital (now Montreal Children's Hospital) intended for 130 patients and seventy-eight nurses on eight floors, designed by hospital specialist J. Cecil McDougall. But by then other Montreal hospitals were also offering private accommodation, so that by the time the MGH pavilion was built, it was no longer in demand. The opening was delayed and three floors remained unfinished.[3]

Every aspect of the architecture of private patients' pavilions stressed separation and differentiation. This concern extended from the siting of the building, which was almost always freestanding, at some distance from an older hospital complex, to the details and finishes of individual rooms. As already mentioned, at the Royal Victoria, the Ross Pavilion was located up Mount Royal to the northwest of the 1893 hospital; this ensured that the 130 wealthy patients for whom the building was intended would have few close encounters with less fortunate patients. This purposeful site planning also meant that the Ross could have a completely independent entry sequence from the rest of the hospital.

Many landscape features of the Ross Pavilion signaled its status as a place for wealthier patients, including a sophisticated formal garden and teahouse planned for its rear, and a special parking court for ambulances (Figure 2.2). Associated with recreation and leisure, such features were commonly found behind larger houses and mansions; their link with the health benefits of ambulation, sunshine, and fresh air, too, made them especially appropriate features for a private patients' pavilion.

Despite the degree of separation afforded by Stevens and Lee's site planning of the Ross Memorial Pavilion, some means of interior connection to the main hospital for staff serving paying patients remained necessary. Given the steep site on the slopes of Mount Royal, this problem was solved with a sophisticated and costly tunnel. The main floor of the Ross is one hundred feet above the floor of the Snell building; the tunnel

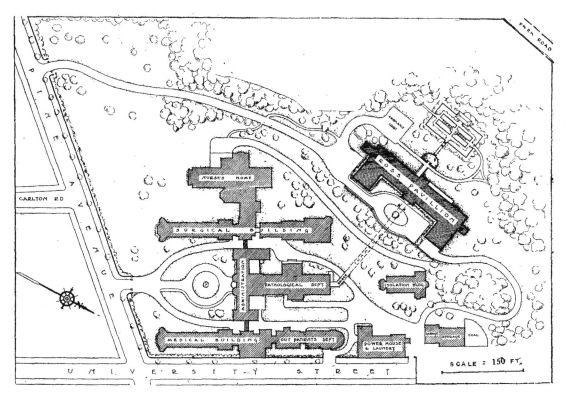

FIGURE 2.2. This site plan shows the garden and teahouse, features commonly associated with domestic architecture.

reached from the second floor of the older hospital, at the back of the Pathology Department, crossed a bridge, and then, with a grade of 5 percent, reached the new elevator
shafts and staircase fifty feet below the main floor of the Ross. Such was the cost of
appearing to be separate, while remaining invisibly connected.

Paying patients' whole experience of the landscape subtly underlined the building's
position at the top, literally and economically, of the hospital. The Ross was purpose-
fully located about one thousand feet above a separate entrance to the site on Pine Avenue.
This assured discretion and seclusion for its class-conscious patients, but also afforded
them fabulous views. Not surprisingly, the entrance to the site from the street (Figure
2.3) was marked by heavy wrought iron gates one might expect to find at a mansion. The
winding driveway climbed several hundred feet to the new hospital, offering changing,
picturesque views of the Victorian building and the bustling commercialized city, before
arrival at the Ross Pavilion itself, a five-story, U-shaped block with an imposing central
tower. The drive then terminated in an elegant oval at the hospital's front door, on its east
side, allowing automobiles and carriages to exit the site in a single, flowing swoop.

Patients of the Ross Pavilion entered the building from the west or rear side, on
the second floor. Here a specially designed park assured that they were "relieved of the

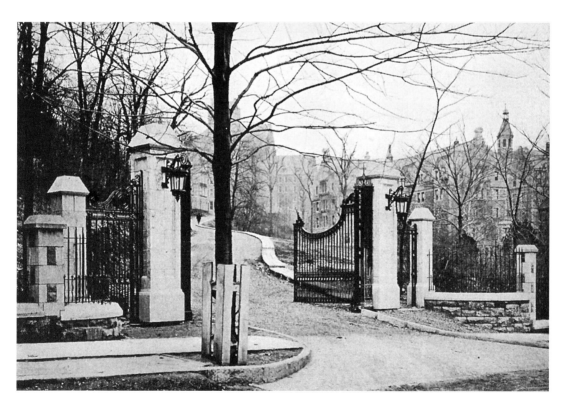

FIGURE 2.3. The elegant entrance gate for automobiles signaled the distinct status of the Ross
Memorial Pavilion, Royal Victoria Hospital.

disturbing noises from the street or from the main hospital buildings."[4] Indeed, the park was designed so that the main buildings of the hospital would be entirely invisible from this location.

Even traces of the building's mechanical systems were concealed from patients who paid for their stays, cloaked in the "false" forms of the building's medieval revival style. The elevator, fans, and ventilation equipment were housed in the hospital's monumental central tower, which overlooked the entrance for patients. Small-scale technologies were hidden, too. The central radiator intended to heat the hospital's generous entry lobby, for instance, was cloaked in a pedestal of marble and oak, with bronze grills, surmounted by a small, illuminated fountain.

The architecture of the Ross, like that of other private patients pavilions, is heaped with domestic ideology. The overall image of the building, with its thick limestone walls and soaring tower (complete with machicolations and four tiny turrets), recalled medieval castles, like the Snell building, which clearly inspired it. But additional references to contemporary upper-class houses and hotels were legible in the building's details. The Ross had thirty suites of two rooms, complete with bath and private balcony; many suites with baths; and large private rooms with baths adjoining. Patients who were considered particularly noisy used two rooms and a bath on the attic floor.[5] Compared to the Snell-designed building, where patients commonly shared a ward with thirty others, the Ross placed a premium on privacy and solitude.

Even at the time, the comparison of these secluded pavilions with hotels was unavoidable. The lobby of the Ross was frequently weighed against the entry spaces of luxurious hotels. Some institutions, such as the Toronto General Hospital, tried to use the hotel analogy to their advantage. Its nine-story T. J. Bell Pavilion of 1930, designed by Toronto architects Darling & Pearson, included both a "Hotel Dining Room" and a "Hotel Wing." At the time of its opening, in fact, the building was described by journalists as a "palatial hotel-hospital."[6] *The Canadian Hospital* devoted an entire issue to the project when it opened. "The rotunda into which the visitor enters is suggestive of a palatial and exclusive hotel rather than a hospital," reported the magazine in 1930. "In fact many features usually associated with first class hotels have been incorporated in the Private Patients Pavilion," continued the journalist. These features even included uniformed attendants to direct traffic, fine furniture, and brocade curtains. Lamps shades were embellished with Chinese embroidered silk and walls were paneled in walnut. The rooms for patients at the Bell Pavilion, which ranged in price from four to twelve dollars a day, even boasted overstuffed chairs in "gay chintz," and the new pavilion's telephone switchboard was as big as that serving the entire city of Oshawa.[7]

Luxurious associations continued outside the hospital, too, with explicit references to resort hotel architecture. Parklike grounds—the Ross was surrounded by Frederick Law Olmsted's magnificent Mount Royal Park—played into the middle-class antiurban penchant for wilderness vacations in the late nineteenth and early twentieth centuries.[8] While urban hospitals were unlikely to boast any of the "natural" and/or water features seen to improve health at popular resorts, such as hot springs or access to hiking trails, the picturesque gardens surrounding pavilions like the Ross gave the patients the impression of a trip outside the city.

Hotel and residential imagery as a mechanism disguising the hospital's association with illness appealed to middle-class patients and also pleased their doctors. Physicians benefited in numerous ways from having private patients, beyond monetary gain. Stevens described the Ross medical treatment department as one that provided the physician "greater opportunities for his work than are provided in the majority of medical institutions."[9] Perhaps he meant that the new buildings provided a choice of therapies, as Stevens illustrated his point with a large-scale plan of the south end of the Ross's first floor, which showed the spaces provided for hydrotherapy, as well as light therapy, massage, and hot and cold packs.

An up-to-date surgical suite was an important part of this package. Stevens called the surgical department at the Ross Pavilion the "most complete."[10] Located on the fifth floor, in the north end of the building, the surgical wing included two large operating rooms. Stevens was particularly proud of the illumination and ventilation of the Ross surgical suite: "entirely indirect, no lighting fixture being in the operating room, but all concealed behind the glazed ceiling."[11] Radiators in the operating room were sandwiched between the outside window and a glass wall, open at the top. This allowed both light and heated, fresh air to enter the room. Two large-scale sections of the Ross arrangement (Figure 2.4) were included in *The American Hospital of the Twentieth Century*.

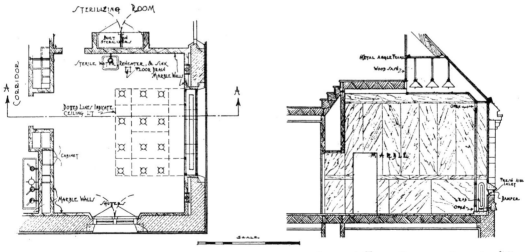

FIGURE 2.4. The surgical suite attracted paying patients to the hospital and justified the hiring of specialists like Stevens.

At a time when the practice of surgery was seen as a particularly scientific feature of hospitals, the transformation of the old-fashioned operating theater into the operating suite signaled the rise of surgery. The interwar suite as a surgical space is very different from the 1893 theater we saw in chapter 1: now the operating room is embedded in the building, though always at one end or on top. In this new type of surgical arrangement the room for surgery is part of a suite of smaller spaces. Stevens's plan shows it included two large operating rooms, as well as surgeons' sitting rooms, two anesthesia rooms, and workrooms. There are no spectators, and certainly the surgery has no direct entry from the exterior as it did in 1893.[12]

Architects doubled and layered materials in order to maximize discretion. The Ross Pavilion had double floors, double partitions, and double windows. Each patient room had two doors; floors of the patient rooms were linoleum, while the corridors were lined with cork. And every patient was provided with all the comforts of home, literally: lavatory, mirror, semidirect ceiling light, portable bedside light, phone connection, and a nurses' call system that resembled the bells typically used to summon domestic staff. Ventilation of the rooms was through individual clothes cupboards, ensuring that the contents of cupboards were thoroughly aired at the same time.

Outpatients

The counterpoint to the private patients pavilion in the construction of the modern hospital was the provision of new facilities for outpatients. The outpatient department, also known as the outdoor, sustained the hospital's mission to serve the poor, since here the hospital treated patients who could not afford to pay for doctors or for accommodation in the wards. As Harvey Agnew showed in his fine, detailed memoir of hospitals from 1920 to 1970, this benevolent role of the Canadian hospital continued well into the 1940s and 1950s. Municipal and provincial governments paid fees to hospitals based on the number of indigents they accommodated, complementing the support they received from individuals and volunteers.[13] The outpatients' plight, then, the reason they were outdoor rather than indoor patients, was determined as much by their social class as by their medical condition.[14]

Not surprisingly, the architecture of the outpatient department was opposite to the private patients pavilion in every possible way. While the private patients department was typically located at some distance from the main hospital, the outpatients department was frequently accommodated within the main building. A Stevens trademark, in fact, was the location of outpatient departments in the basement of the older hospital. So while paying patients literally traveled "upward" to their quarters, poorer outpatients descended.

And while private patients were offered privacy and seclusion, outpatient departments were nearly always congested. The only "separate" feature of the modern outpatient department was a separate entrance, which, while providing a special place of entry for poorer patients, also served to exclude them from the main entry to the hospital. And like the vertical relationship established between the wealthy patients at the Ross, who literally looked down on their poorer fellow patients, the main hospital door was often "above" that intended for outpatients. Such was the case at the Stevens-designed Ottawa Civic Hospital, where there was considerable objection to Stevens's design for outpatient stairs going down. Despite its rather unpretentious setting, the outpatient department continued to fulfill an important symbolic function: proof that the hospital continued to be a charitable organization for the benefit of the sick poor. As such, outpatient departments were a significant meeting place between the general public and medical technology, often tied into public health programs (such as anti-venereal disease clinics). And in the interwar period, one of the ways that new groups of poor patients entered the hospital was as outpatients. There the poor encountered diagnostic testing and measuring of medical problems (including minor surgery, regular checkups, lab tests, X-rays) much more intensely than they probably did on the wards.

By the late 1920s, many hospitals were constructing separate outpatient departments and remodeling existing buildings. *The Modern Hospital* conducted a survey in 1926. Of 500 nonteaching hospitals reporting to the magazine, 34 had built new outpatient buildings during 1923 and 1924; 85 had new buildings projected; in 76, some new construction had been made; 83 had assigned more space to the outpatient departments without construction; and in 87, improvements in the department were planned but not yet undertaken.[15]

Stevens remodeled the former four-story pathology department at the Royal Victoria for outpatients in 1922.[16] Although this department was not in the basement, its strategic location along University Street, just north of Snell's original medical wing, meant that it was in close proximity to the hospital's most industrial sectors: the powerhouse, laundry, and garage. This work-a-day context links outpatient facilities to dispensaries in poor neighborhoods. Many of the so-called medical dispensaries in Montreal occupied shop-front spaces. They dispensed medicine and were associated with the doctors and visiting nurses who made home visits to poor patients. As will be discussed in chapter 3, this western edge of the hospital was also home to the more "scientific," masculine sectors of the institution, such as pathology and neurology. Obstetrical patients and student nurses were kept as far away from poor patients as possible on most sites.

At the heart of nearly every Stevens outpatient department design was a generous waiting room. Resembling the arrival halls of railway stations, these large spaces often included bench seating and vaulted ceilings.[17] Outpatient departments thus drew inspiration from the public architecture of the city, rather than the cozy world of the home or the luxurious, leisure-based realm of the grand hotel, reflecting their continuing roles as places open to a wide public. The bench seating is a further example (in addition to location and entry sequence) of how the material culture of the outpatient department differed from the mandate of separation that we saw in private patients pavilions: poor families huddled next to each other on benches without any barrier (i.e., not even the arm of a chair) between them. This bench seating, where outpatients sat next to strangers without separation, echoed the public wards in which acoustical, visual, and tactile privacy was minimal.

In his ideal plan for a rectangular outpatient department, published in *The American Hospital of the Twentieth Century*, the waiting room is a grand, two-story space with galleries on the second floor.[18] The architect said the separate building for outpatients should not be wider than thirty-six to forty feet, and preferably L-shaped. Stevens's outpatient departments also followed regional trends. In institutions he planned for the southern states, for example, such as the Macon City Hospital, in Macon, Georgia, the outpatient departments had separate waiting rooms (and entrances) for "coloreds" and "whites," exactly like train stations and other public places in which people waited.

OBSTETRICAL PATIENTS

These same spatial urges to be separate, yet together, to reserve the top for the rich and the basement for the poor, marked the new architecture designed for female patients, the maternity hospital. From 1918 to 1940, the number of North American women giving birth in hospitals, rather than at home, grew astronomically. By 1940, 92 percent of all live births took place in the hospital in at least one major Canadian urban center.[19] By 1960, specialists managed nearly 100 percent of deliveries in American hospitals.[20] This massive transformation of the hospital as the place of birth had remarkably little effect on the shockingly high infant and maternal mortality rates that inspired it; the presence of thousands of pregnant women, however, had a profound impact on the development of hospital architecture. "During the interwar period and the following years, the science of obstetrics took pride of place," summarizes Wendy Mitchinson in her classic history of childbirth in Canada.[21]

Designed by Stevens for the Royal Vic in 1926, the maternity pavilion was located high on the site, next to the Ross Memorial Pavilion. Given the clear division by social class we observed in the paying patients pavilion typology, it is not surprising that private obstetrical patients occupied the uppermost floors; they entered the building from their own private entrance, facing Mount Royal on the first floor of the building, like the patients entry at the Ross. This entrance for paying female patients was originally reached by a private road, and the lobby was sumptuously finished in wood paneling. A photo published in *The Canadian Hospital* the same year as the building opened shows the elegant entry sequence designed for paying patients (Figure 2.5). Although the photograph is labeled "vestibule," it depicts the space described on Stevens's plans as "entry hall." Directly on axis with the entry was a view through the waiting room windows to the rest of the hospital, the university campus, and the commercial core of Montreal, evidence of its position of privilege.

Poorer patients, on the other hand, entered the building virtually underground (fifty-six feet below paying patients), at the University Street entrance, which was accessible by streetcar. Like the general outpatient department, it was perilously close to the hospital's powerhouse, laundry, and garage. The level intended for public patients was that labeled the second floor by Stevens (Figure 2.6). The two wards here, located at both ends of the plan and giving onto generous solaria, held sixteen patients, in four-bed cubicles (partitions were of hardwood and seven feet tall). A photograph of the ward shows the arrangement of beds and also a sink and mirror on the column, presumably shared by the patients in the ward (Figure 2.7).

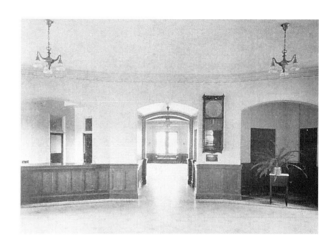

FIGURE 2.5. The aligned doorways of the elegant lobby of the Royal Victoria Montreal Maternity Hospital offered spectacular views of Montreal.

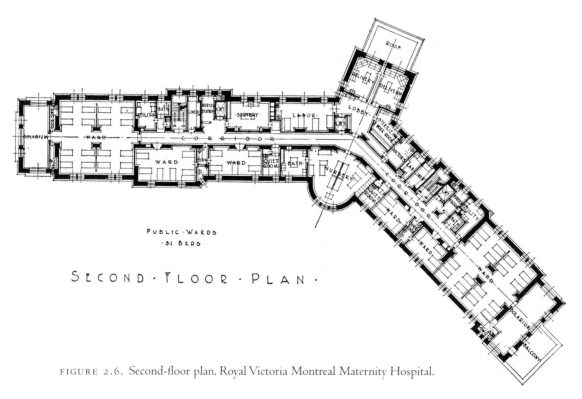

FIGURE 2.6. Second-floor plan, Royal Victoria Montreal Maternity Hospital.

In terms of these vertical relationships, then, the new hospital for women was a model of the city, the entire hospital, and other modern structures.[22] Wealthier patients occupied the uppermost levels, literally looking down on the sick poor, in the same way that expensive homes in Montreal and elsewhere took the loftiest sites, at considerable distance from industrial sectors. The cross section of interwar hospitals, indeed, resembled the vertical progression in luxury ships like the *Titanic*, designed contemporaneously to the Ross, where the third-class berths were located well below the other quarters.

An unusual and revealing source, a description by hospital supervisor Caroline Barrett, outlines a typical stay at the women's pavilion by a public obstetrical patient in 1932. It provides remarkable detail about the way a typical patient moved through such structures, confirming how they operated as two buildings in one.[23] After repeated visits to the hospital clinic, a woman in labor would be taken directly to the admission room, where a nurse would prepare her for an examination. These facilities were located one level above the public entry.[24] As if to compensate for its subterranean location, Stevens provided outpatients with a handsome, sky-lit waiting room (Figure 2.8), complete with four

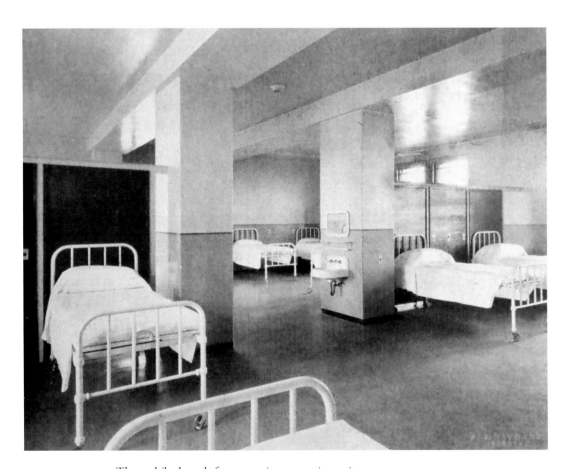

FIGURE 2.7. The multibed wards for nonpaying maternity patients.

classical columns. True to form, however, the seating was eight straight-backed benches. From here, the patient would then move to a dedicated labor room (second floor), where she would be watched until delivery. After delivery (in the room on the second floor), the public patient would remain for one hour, and then be moved to the ward. If feverish, she would be transferred to the isolation department. The typical length of stay of a maternity patient in 1930 was ten days.[25] Presumably she would exit the building the way she entered, by what Stevens referred to as the subground and tunnel levels (Figure 2.9). It was thus unlikely that middle-class and working-class female patients' paths would ever cross in the modern maternity hospital, just as first-class and third-class passengers on ships like the *Titanic* would not come into contact.

This careful separation of paying and nonpaying patients was standard in the inter-war period. Stevens returned to the overall plan of the building, which he called the "bent angle plan," on other steep sites. He used it for the 165-bed Lying-in Hospital in Providence, Rhode Island (Figure 2.10).[26] This V-shaped, long and narrow, double-loaded corridor arrangement maximized light and air. At the apex of the wings were

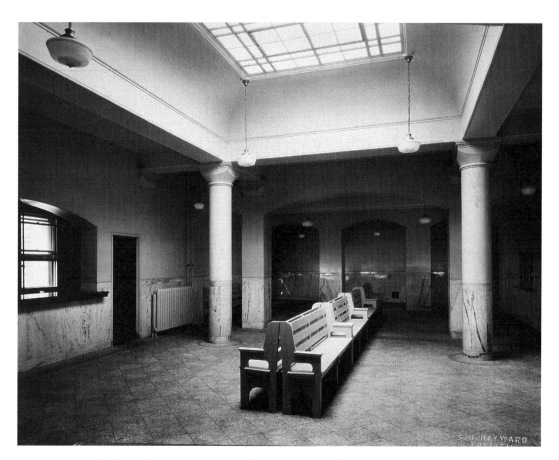

FIGURE 2.8. Outpatients' waiting room with benches and skylight.

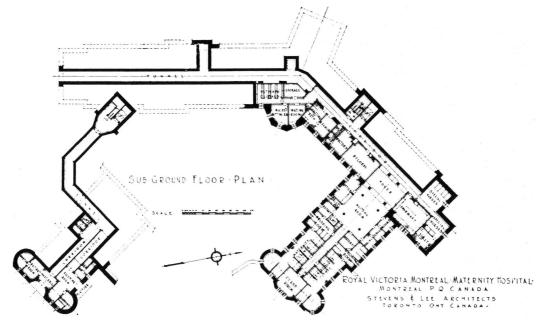

OUT-PATIENT DEPARTMENT

FIGURE 2.9. The entry sequence for poorer patients at the Royal Victoria Montreal Maternity Hospital was subterranean.

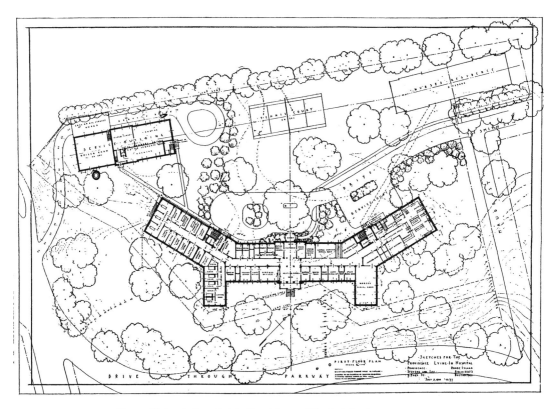

FIGURE 2.10. Plan of lying-in hospital in Providence, Rhode Island.

located major public spaces: kitchen, waiting room on the first-floor (middle-class) level, nurseries for two floors above this, ward, workroom, and finally a living room for nurses (one hundred nurses lived in the building). A photograph of the nurses' living room shows it furnished in relatively simple dark leather armchairs and couches (Figure 2.11). A wooden table with flowers is at the center of the room. Above the elaborate lobby were delivery rooms for public patients, small wards, and a surgical amphitheater with skylight (Figure 2.12). The accommodation for patients occupied the rooms along the corridors. The new hospital was built to accommodate 208 patients in total (obstetrics: public, 61; private, 43; gynecology: public, 46; private, 48; isolation, 10).

Like its immediate neighbor, the Ross Pavilion, Stevens's maternity pavilion (Figure 2.13) looked like an old castle from the exterior. It, too, boasted a central tower, crowning the apex of the angle, rather than marking the building's entrance. The tower's clock lent the building a considerable civic presence. Perhaps as a mark of resistance to the medicalization of childbirth, Stevens himself said that maternity hospitals, among specialized buildings, "should have the social element emphasized; that is, there should be

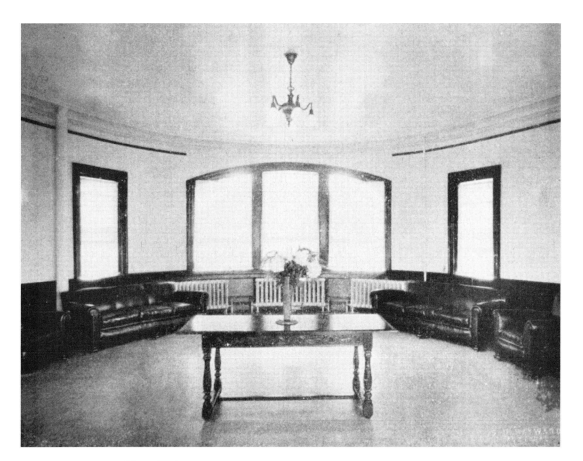

FIGURE 2.11. Nurses' living room.

larger social halls, more lounging space."[27] He emphasized the significance of portraying a "homelike" atmosphere, perhaps in an effort to attract paying patients, like the Ross, but also because he saw childbirth as "a natural function and a part of the home life."

Mitchinson has identified this perspective on birth as a natural event as one of two divisive views on childbirth in the early twentieth century.[28] It is ironic that the opposing view, which positioned childbirth as a pathological event, was what gave real impetus to the construction of maternity hospitals. Childbirth as a pathological event justified the extensive record keeping and observation that the new hospitals supported. Physicians offered women "vigilance and intervention" as part of a hospital birth; the experience also offered them something of an escape from the responsibilities of life at home.[29]

Home births, which dominated the era before World War I, were inconvenient for physicians, too. Travel ate up precious time for doctors; carrying heavy equipment for use during deliveries was difficult. Bedrooms and houses in general were not set up

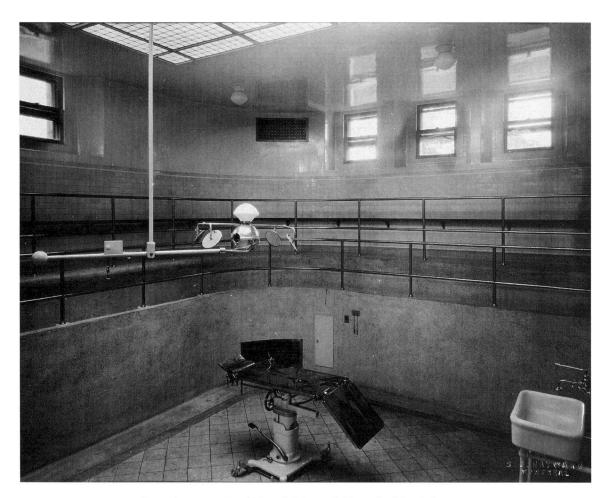

FIGURE 2.12. Operating room, Royal Victoria Montreal Maternity Hospital.

for childbirth, and doctors increasingly relied on a team of colleagues, especially nurses, who couldn't always be present during home deliveries. Husbands and family members, reported doctors, often got in the way.[30] Specialized maternity hospitals solved all these problems. They centralized experts and equipment, offered custom, aseptic delivery rooms, and kept out husbands and other children. Teams of highly specialized nurses and doctors repeated the procedure over and over, working toward predictable results. Careful records were kept, especially regarding the timing of labor, helping obstetricians to predict the ways delivery might go by developing a model of "normal" birth.

The residential image of the interwar maternity hospital countered or at least offset the tensions between understanding birth as a natural or a pathological event. Those who saw birth as a natural event, like Stevens himself, could point to fine wood paneling, tile floors, fireplaces, oil paintings, traditional furniture, and printed textiles in the building. To them the maternity building was just like a grand mansion, only cleaner and quieter. The architect's insistence on a domestic ambience in the hospital made sense in an era when maternity stays were typically ten to twelve days. The inclusion of lounges in the building program for maternity pavilions, for example, shows how architecture served as a tool in the modern concept of recuperation from birth. Lounges with comfortable

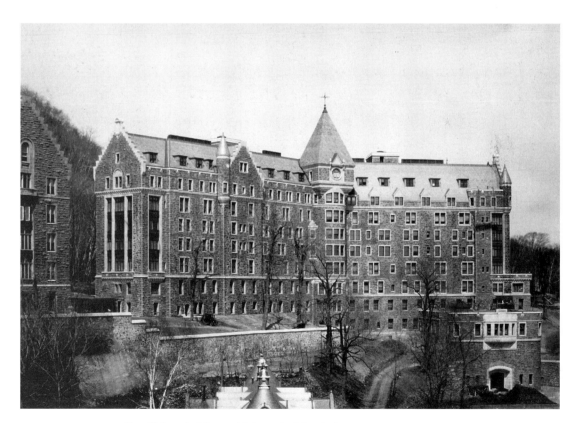

FIGURE 2.13. Royal Victoria Montreal Maternity Hospital.

furniture and spectacular views invited expectant and recovering mothers to relax, even recline, and to socialize with other patients. As a transitional space between the solitude of the private room and the return to life at home, maternity lounges offered middle-class patients quiet, comfortable space in which to heal. If birth was indeed pathological, as hospital physicians argued, or anything like surgery, as its increasingly standardized procedures suggested, then it followed that a period of healing was required. The association with domestic architecture, according to Stevens, was especially important in the design of the maternity hospital's entrance. "The entrance to the hospital should be indicative of hospitality and should present a homelike welcome to the would-be guest," he said in 1922. "This should be a home where the expectant mother may enter as she would her own home, with a feeling of safety and comfort."

To adherents of birth as a pathological moment, however, the maternity pavilion offered more than these comforting touches. Patients were "prepped" for delivery like surgery patients; genitalia were scrubbed and shaved. Pain relief was available to delivering women, much more readily than it had been at home. Just as the procedures surrounding birth borrowed from the techniques of modern surgery, delivery rooms resembled operating rooms; the furniture was metal, wheeled, and easily cleaned. All surfaces were tiled and corners were rounded, in order not to harbor dust and germs. Teams of experts were ready for anything.

The basic division of wealthy women on top and poorer women down below was the central idea behind the building's organization. Women who paid for their stays benefited from the magnificent views afforded from Mount Royal, the quiet and the fresh air available hundreds of feet above the street. Reviews of the building following its opening emphasize (and perhaps exaggerate) the importance of its views:

> The Royal Victoria Montreal Maternity Hospital stands, therefore, to-day, upon probably one of the most picturesque sites possessed by any institution in the world. Nestled upon the slopes of historic Mount Royal, it is situated in the centre of the second oldest city upon the North American continent. The mighty St. Lawrence River runs practically past its front door. The horizon, extending southward fully twenty-five miles, is carried to the very foothills of the Adirondack Range.[31]

Many of the same technologies afforded to paying patients at the Ross were also made available to female paying patients in this new building, including sophisticated ventilation, an elaborate call system and locating signal, telephone wiring, special night-lights, wiring for electrocardiograph, fountains with fresh sterile drinking water, microleveling elevators, and soundproofing.[32]

Two photographs of private rooms in the maternity hospital illustrate the ways in which the rooms were furnished. The new women's hospital was frequently featured in advertisements for flooring (see Figure 5.6).[33] An advertisement for rubberized flooring (Figure 2.14) features a room with a single metal bed, two wooden armchairs, and a

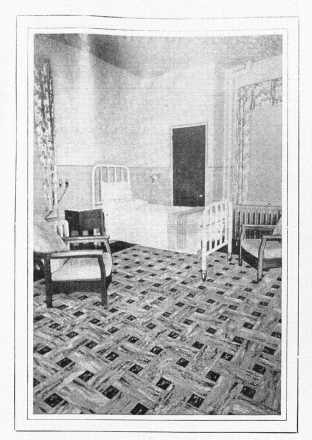
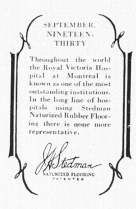
FIGURE 2.14. Rubberized flooring was associated with the modern hospital.

bedside table. The door in the photograph may be an internal connection to a nurses'
room. An archival photograph (Figure 2.15) shows a slightly less luxurious arrangement,
with a metal bed in the room's corner, a regular chair and an armchair, a bedside table,
and a dresser with a mirror. Again, there is a door that plans show is some sort of interior connection.

Obstetrical patients constituted a new and significant user group of the interwar
hospital, as is clear from the monumental and specialized buildings designed for them.
Do female patients merit analysis beyond the theme of obstetrics? From an architectural
perspective they do not, even in the face of a notable increase in numbers. While the late-
nineteenth-century hospital was essentially an institution for sick, poor young men—
about 80 percent of patients fit that description—the interwar hospital attracted more
women. But it was only in maternity pavilions and later in nurses' residences that hospital experts saw the need to separate women and to offer them a distinct architectural
experience. As we will see in chapter 3, the home for nurses, like the maternity pavilion,
engaged domestic imagery to attract, retain, and comfort middle-class women.

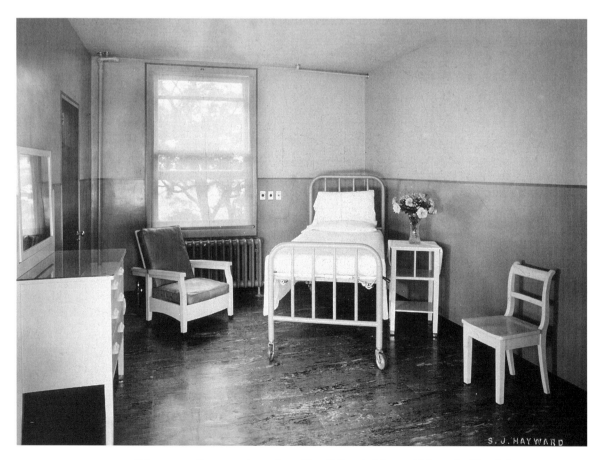

FIGURE 2.15. Private room for maternity patients, Royal Victoria Montreal Maternity Hospital, 1926.

CHILDREN

The accommodation for children within the nineteenth-century general hospital illustrates how and why separate, purpose-built pavilions for children were considered unnecessary in Montreal as the nineteenth century drew to a close. At Snell's Royal Victoria Hospital, for example, young patients were mostly integrated with others in the rather sprawling, pavilion-plan structure.[34] (As discussed in chapter 1, the most prominent features of the design by British architect Henry Saxon Snell were the large, open "Nightingale" wards, which housed surgical and medical patients on either side of a central administration block, to which they were minimally connected.) Apart from a dedicated children's surgical ward in a short extension behind the general surgical wards, young patients were accorded no special spaces in the new building.[35] Snell's published plan (see Figure 1.21) of the main floor, which differs slightly from the way the building was eventually constructed, makes no reference to children.

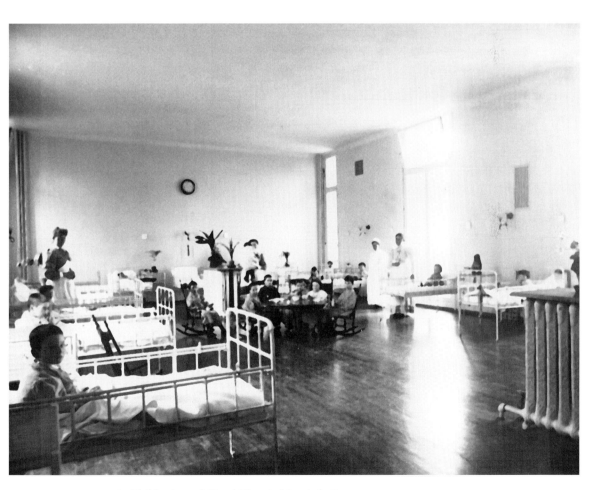

FIGURE 2.16. Children's ward, Royal Victoria Hospital, 1894.

They were also, it seems, rarely photographed. Few photographs have survived illustrating the spaces occupied by children at the Royal Victoria, and only one of these actually shows children. William Notman's stunning photograph of 1894 (Figure 2.16) reveals one end of a pavilion-style ward, with four adult women, twelve beds, and seventeen children. The clock, plants, and marble-topped radiators are identical to those found in the adult wards. Not surprisingly, Notman captured the children's ward with its windows open, illustrating contemporary preoccupations with fresh air. What differentiates this ward from others of the hospital is the recreational use of the space between the radiators. Notman's photo shows six children, seated in small rockers, enjoying "tea" with a tiny tea service at a table specially scaled for them.

Minor adjustments occurred in the accommodation of children as the hospital developed over the next fifteen years or so, indicating the growing importance of child patients as a special group. In 1907, for example, pediatrics was given its own ward mostly for patients recovering from minor surgery, like the removal of tonsils. In 1919, the children's medical ward was relocated to Ward N, where it remained for the next four decades.[36] A photograph of Ward N (Figure 2.17) shows beds on only one side of the room; apart from this arrangement, the scale of the beds, and the toy dog in the photo,

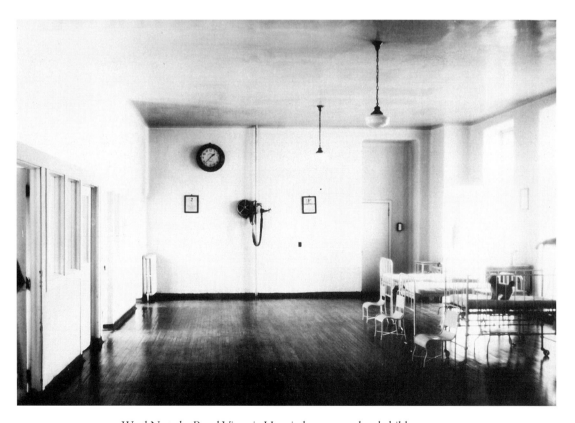

FIGURE 2.17. Ward N at the Royal Victoria Hospital accommodated children.

the space differs little from the adult wards at the hospital. In short, the visual evidence, from the time the hospital opened in 1893, shows that children were treated (spatially) like the other patients who stayed at the new hospital, except, crucially, they were given opportunity and spaces for play.

During the same era, Toronto's sick children were more visible in the cultural landscape of the city. They occupied a purpose-built facility for children as early as 1891. Designed by Frank Darling and S. G. Curry, who had designed Toronto's Home for Incurables a decade earlier, the Victoria Hospital for Sick Children (Figure 2.18) was a large Romanesque Revival block, located amidst the city's tenements on College Street. Its steeply pitched roofs, like those of the Royal Victoria in Montreal, lent the institution an aristocratic air, conjuring up obvious associations with castles, but also resembling the elaborate railway hotels constructed across Canada at this time, such as the Château Laurier in Ottawa and the Château Frontenac in Quebec City.[37]

The Victoria Hospital for Sick Children (later the Hospital for Sick Children), founded in 1875, was typical of other pioneering institutions in that it combined the needs of medical science with an equally strong drive for social and moral amelioration, organized by benevolent, middle-class women. The world's first hospital for children was the Hôpital des Enfants Malades in Paris in 1802. London's celebrated Hospital for Sick Children in Great Ormond Street opened in 1852. The first American hospital for children

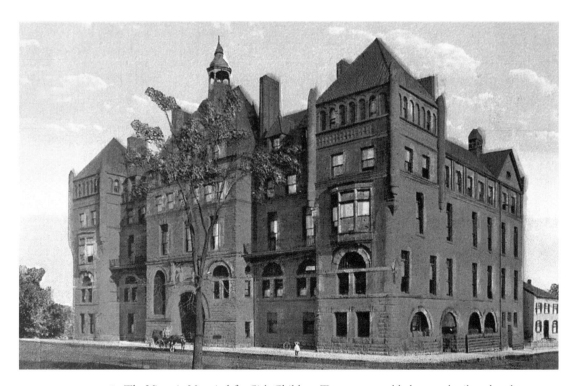

FIGURE 2.18. The Victoria Hospital for Sick Children, Toronto, resembled a grand railway hotel.

was New York's in 1854.[38] By 1890, according to historian David C. Sloane, there were thirty children's hospitals in the United States. Most of these early buildings relied on domestic ideology to express the benevolent part of its dual mission, appearing to be a "big house" that would provide poor, sick children with both protection and a surrogate family atmosphere.[39] This semblance of domesticity, accomplished largely through the hospital's massing, roof type, materials, scale, decoration, plan, and furniture, also related it to reform buildings like settlement houses. These, too, were controlled by women and were intended to improve the lives of working-class kids through various educational initiatives.[40]

In general terms, the plan (Figure 2.19) of Toronto's Victoria Hospital for Sick Children was similar to the Royal Victoria Hospital; it was an E-shaped mass with a central entry on the north and open wards reaching south. Smaller wards were located along the College Street elevation, separated by pantries and doctors' rooms. The only features in the plan that distinguished the hospital for children from that for adults were a playground for convalescent children and a conservatory, in the middle arm of the E on the second floor. Play and fresh air were thus fundamental to its mandate.[41]

It was mostly due to the complications of observing and isolating children in regular wards that the need for separate children's pavilions was articulated. The influential German pediatricians Carl Rauchfuss in 1877 and, a half-century later, Emil Freed in 1928 cited the need to isolate patients with infectious diseases as the compelling reason for separate children's hospitals.[42] But there were reasons for and against this isolationist approach. Both for infant feeding and social reasons, for instance, adults and newborns needed to be accommodated together. The support for the specialist children's hospital thus developed only slowly. As late as 1910, Charles Butler would still claim that "the Children's Hospital as a separate institution is a recent development in the United States."[43] Five years later, Dr. Henry Dwight Chapin wrote against the hospitalization of infants, arguing that "[t]he best conditions for the infant thus require a home and a mother." "I do not believe," he wrote, "that the multiplication of infant's hospitals through the country should be encouraged."[44]

Stevens and Lee designed several early children's hospitals and were important figures in the development of the type. In *The American Hospital of the Twentieth Century,* Stevens addressed this tricky question of the separation of children in the general hospital. Noting the need to isolate them from the general patient population because of the relative high frequency of communicable diseases among the young, Stevens recommended a special observation ward for children, separated from other patient areas by screens. At the same time, however, he reminded readers that sick children, unlike most adults, benefited from the company of others. A glass screen (Figure 2.20) separating every three to four beds, in wards not larger than sixteen to twenty beds, was ideal in his opinion.[45]

In a typically immodest way, Stevens considered his own firm's design for the Isolation Pavilion of the Toronto Hospital for Sick Children of 1912 a model children's hospital, perhaps because it was based on the Pasteur Institute in Paris.[46] As will be discussed in the conclusion, seeing the famous French institution had a profound effect on the young

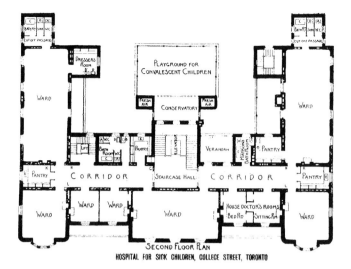

SECOND FLOOR PLAN
HOSPITAL FOR SICK CHILDREN, COLLEGE STREET, TORONTO

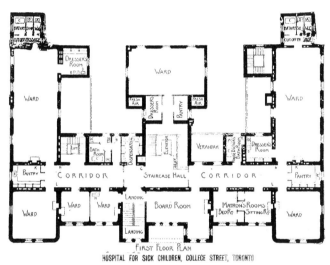

FIRST FLOOR PLAN
HOSPITAL FOR SICK CHILDREN, COLLEGE STREET, TORONTO

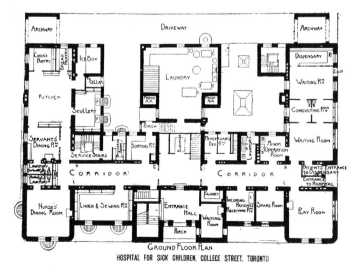

FIGURE 2.19.
The floor plans of the
Victoria Hospital for
Sick Children maximize
air and light.

GROUND FLOOR PLAN
HOSPITAL FOR SICK CHILDREN, COLLEGE STREET, TORONTO

American architect. Stevens designed glass cubicles for isolating contagious patients (an arrangement known among hospital designers and consultants as "the Pasteur principle"), and a narrow, continuous balcony surrounding the building, a feature intended to accommodate visiting friends and family.

The interior of Stevens and Lee's pavilion illustrates the influence of the Paris hospital. A photograph of the Toronto hospital published in *The American Hospital of the Twentieth Century* shows a view down the interior corridor of the isolation building at Toronto's Hospital for Sick Children (Figure 2.21). The dividing walls (between hall and rooms, and between rooms and rooms) are plate glass held by a system of metal framing, extending from floor to ceiling. The overall aesthetic was one of transparency, lightness, and modularity, architectural qualities associated with Modernism, and a stark contrast to the thick masonry walls of Darling and Curry's 1891 chateauesque building.[47] A second, particularly scientific feature of these early-twentieth-century children's hospitals was the provision of space intended for the pasteurization of milk. Stevens included a photograph of the Toronto hospital's pasteurizing room (Figure 2.22) in his book, as well

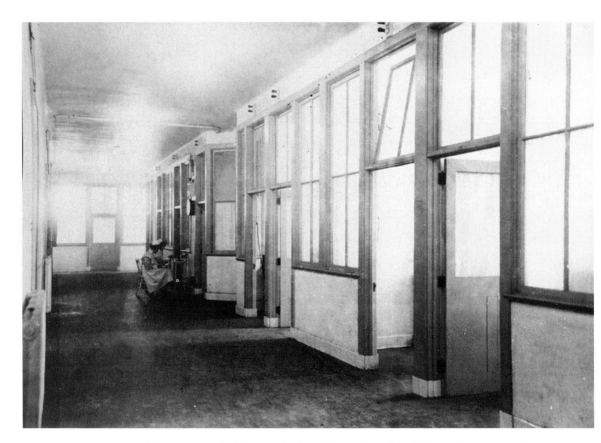

FIGURE 2.20. Glass screens at Hôpital Ste-Justine, Montreal, combined the need for segregation and surveillance.

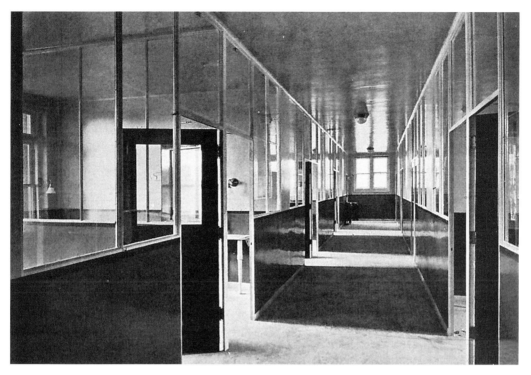

FIGURE 2.21. This view down an interior corridor of the Isolation Pavilion in Toronto's Hospital for Sick Children showcases the transparency of glass partitions.

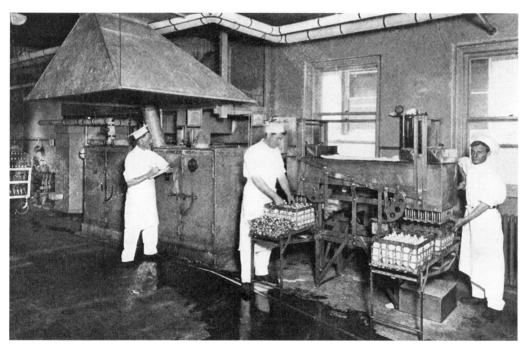

FIGURE 2.22. A pasteurizing room was a distinct feature of children's hospitals. Hospital for Sick Children, Toronto.

as the plan of the children's hospital he designed for Halifax. The Toronto hospital, according to Stevens, had the most "complete" plant for the pasteurization of milk for an institution of its size, fulfilling its own demand as well as providing for outpatient distribution.[48]

Apart from these two decidedly modern features (cubicles and milk rooms), however, purpose-built hospitals for children in the first half of the twentieth century provided few technologies or medical spaces different from those of the general hospitals, reflecting the ambiguous relationship of pediatrics to other medical specialties.[49] Pediatrican Alton Goldbloom, for example, described Montreal's Children's Memorial Hospital in 1920 as "inactive" and "isolated" (especially in winter), with "few facilities for special treatment."[50] Milk rooms were widely distributed outside of children's hospitals. In fact, pediatric care did develop some specialized machinery, notably the incubator.[51] But this technology was used as often in general hospitals as in children's hospitals. And historian Joel D. Howell warns that the existence of a technology does not determine how, where, or when it was used.[52] Still, Goldbloom soon resigned his post at the Montreal General Hospital, believing that "the future of pediatrics in Montreal lay not in the children's departments of the large hospitals, but in the Children's Hospital," which was only gradually becoming "something more than a hospital for crippled children."[53]

Indeed, the central ideas behind the design of the Children's Memorial Hospital in Montreal emphasized lingering, somewhat outdated notions of social reform and maternal benevolence, founded on a nostalgic view of childhood, rather than serving the hospital's newfound scientific orientation. Perhaps the most romantic aspect of the hospital was its site (Figure 2.23). Located across the street from the current Montreal General Hospital and just to the west of the Shriners' Hospital for Crippled Children (designed by Montreal architects J. M. Miller and Hugh Vallance, 1924), the Children's Memorial Hospital occupied the wooded slopes of Mount Royal.[54] It resembled other public institutions ringing the Olmsted-planned picturesque park, notably the Université de Montréal, Notre-Dame cemeteries, and the Royal Victoria Hospital. Part of its benevolent vocation was thus fulfilled by the site, as the hospital was intended to enhance the healing of sick poor kids by removing them from the crowded and damp quarters in which they lived, to the low-density and fresh air of Mount Royal.

As Denise Lemieux has shown in her study of childhood in Quebec literature, this vocation stemmed both from concerns about sanitary conditions of the poor and from a dream of a mythic childhood located somewhere in Quebec's rural origins.[55] A good example is Gabrielle Roy's *The Tin Flute* (1945). In chapter 18, Rose-Anna visits her son Daniel Lacasse, a patient in the Children's Memorial Hospital. The image of the hospital as portrayed in this classic account of working-class urban life is unforgettable. Roy describes the sweep of gracious mansions that surround the hospital's prestigious Cedar Avenue address, and the cheerful light inside the building: the polished floors, the gleaming whiteness, and the abundance of toys for Daniel. But in Roy's account, the hospital has a dark side, too. We feel Rose-Anna's fatigue as she labors up the long, steep climb to reach Daniel on Mount Royal. Rose-Anna feels swallowed up by the hospital's corridors and dismayed at the young nurse's insistence on communicating in English. The emotional climax of Roy's chapter is Rose-Anna's recognition that Daniel has never been so happy.

A major difference between the Royal Victoria Hospital and the Children's Memorial Hospital was in the significance accorded to exterior spaces. Whereas the immediate surroundings of the Royal Victoria Hospital had served only as a picturesque framework to the hospital itself, exterior spaces at the Children's Memorial actually functioned as outdoor wards for patients. Photos show children dressed for both summer and winter weather outside in beds and nurses taking the temperature of patients in the gardens. Some images are clearly of special events, like the shot of Commencement Day that appeared in the hospital's 1912 annual report; others, however, such as one of a nurse with three beds on a walkway outside the hospital (Figure 2.24), are more ambiguous. In both cases, however, the images underline how important the exterior, forested spaces were to the workings of the Children's Memorial Hospital in this period, perhaps a consequence of the hospital's continuing struggle against tuberculosis.

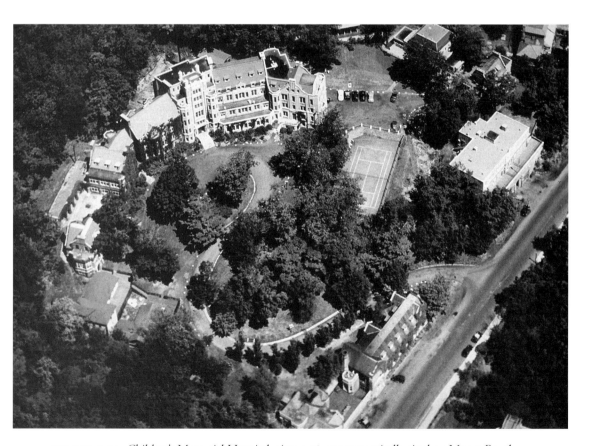

FIGURE 2.23. Children's Memorial Hospital, circa 1936, was romantically sited on Mount Royal.

Outdoor spaces were also a distinctive design feature of the Children's Memorial Hospital master plan. The general arrangement of the site, as drawn by architects David Robertson Brown and Hugh Vallance, was for a series of fourteen pavilions linked by walkways, forming a loop from Cedar Avenue. Directly accessible from the street were the James Carruthers Outpatient Building (1920) and the School (1916). Farther up the hill, at the end of a circular driveway, were the administration building, the Sarah Maxwell Memorial, and the Arnott Cottage (1913). Smaller buildings on the site included the Kiwanis Hut (1924), the Kinmond Cottage (1925), the Judah Memorial Pavilion (1926), a hut for twenty boys with TB (1928), the Forbes Building (1931), the George G. Foster Hut (1932), and the Hazel Fountaine Brown Pavilion (1935).

Another particularly distinctive feature of the Children's Memorial Hospital architecture was that the corridor rooftops (Figure 2.25) also served as wards; tents that functioned as wards were scattered throughout the grounds.[56] A perspective drawing of this unusual corridor type was published on the back of the Children's Memorial Hospital Annual Report in 1919, in the hope that a benefactor would subsidize this "corridor leading from the upper storey of the Hospital to the mountain park . . . [for] the open-air treatment of little children suffering from deforming diseases" such as rickets and tuberculosis of the spine.

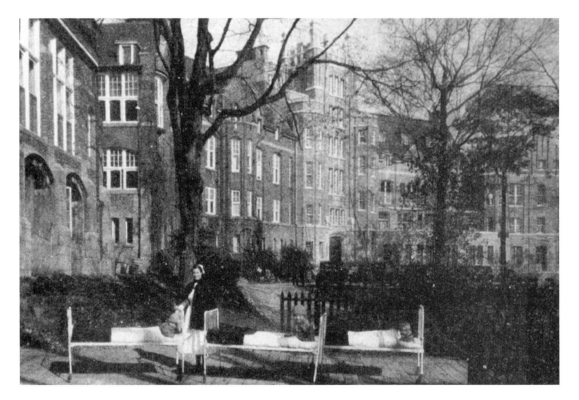

FIGURE 2.24. This nurse "walking" three patients in beds shows the importance of outdoor spaces.

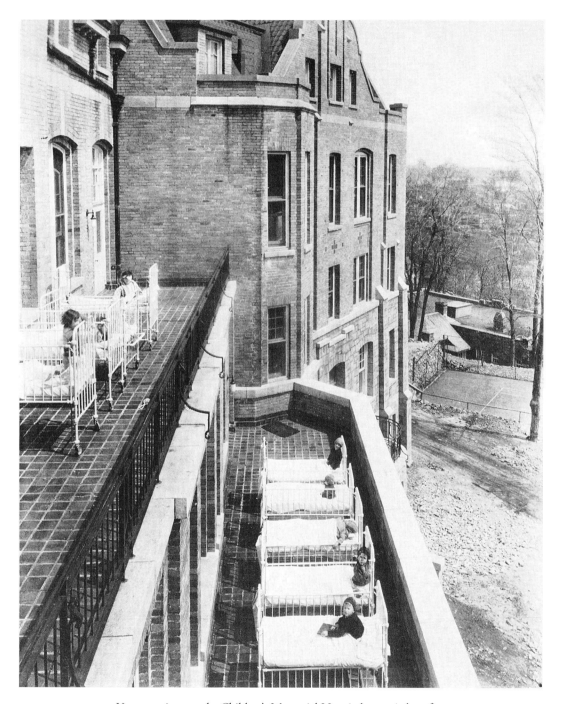

FIGURE 2.25. Young patients at the Children's Memorial Hospital occupied rooftops.

Orthopedics was a second important focus of children's hospitals. In the case of the Children's Memorial Hospital, interior photographs of orthopedic patients show it to be a comparatively nonscientific institution. Photographs show hutlike rooms with visible structure and (sometimes) exposed plumbing (Figure 2.26). While these images may have been taken for the purpose of fund-raising (and thus emphasize the building in need of repair), they also illustrate just how bucolic the buildings were. In fact, the photographs resemble images of overseas hospitals during World War I, both for their emphasis on rehabilitation and for the flimsy, ephemeral appearance of the architecture.

Despite its concentration on children's needs, the architecture of the Children's Memorial Hospital was far from modern. The ensemble was composed of temporary, unheated huts; it had one operating room; its X-ray department was lagging; the outpatients' department was difficult to access; and its school for crippled children suffered from competition from the neighboring Shriners' Hospital. At the Children's Memorial Hospital, even scientific nursing, an indispensable part of the modern medical center as we will see in chapter 3, lagged behind. The training school closed in 1934 as part of the modernization of the nurses' education program at the McGill teaching hospitals. Not until 1931 did the institution have a distinct nurses' residence and not until the 1950s did nurses have their own building.

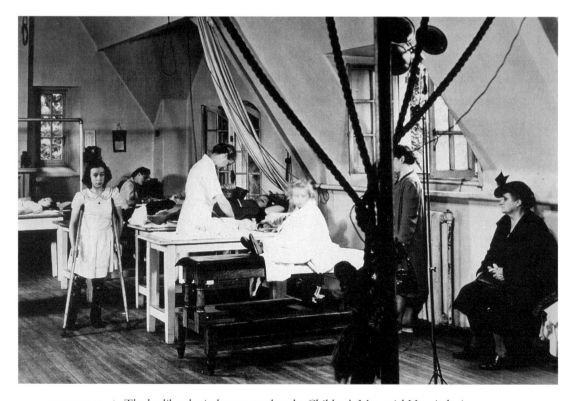

FIGURE 2.26. The hutlike physiotherapy ward at the Children's Memorial Hospital, circa 1942.

Perhaps the continuing significance of outdoor space in the architectural evolution of the Children's Memorial Hospital also derives from its rather ad hoc beginnings. The institution, like many others, first occupied a rented house (1903). Renovations to it cost $400, financed by a sale of homemade goods by Montreal schoolchildren. From January 1904 to May 1905, 122 patients and 195 outpatients were treated there. The patients admitted to the ad hoc quarters suffered from tuberculosis (46), rickets (17), infantile paralysis (5), other paralysis (6), and other diseases (48). The cost of patient care was twenty-eight cents a day, or about 20 percent as much as the daily patient cost at the Royal Victoria Hospital a decade earlier.[57]

Under a new director, in 1936, the hospital attempted to modernize on the model of the technology-oriented (i.e., Stevens type) modern hospital. The ensuing fund-raising campaign publicized images (Figure 2.27) of a hospital designed by emerging hospital specialist J. Cecil McDougall in a self-consciously modern idiom. This was a clear bid to associate the modern children's hospital with modern architecture. The annual reports at this time, too, show a clear transition in style and tone from an earlier romantic view of childhood disease, to the more contemporary, officious, scientific style associated with the general hospital.

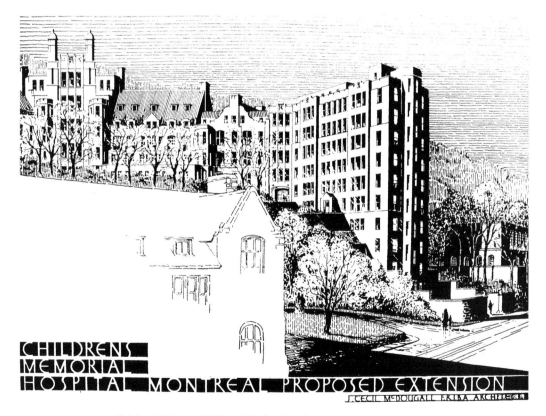

FIGURE 2.27. Children's Memorial Hospital, fund-raising perspective.

The hospital's architecture can be read as evidence of the great difficulty experienced by the hospital in asserting itself as a center of research and teaching, reflected, too, in the struggle for academic recognition of pediatrics. For example, Harold Beveridge Cushing did not convince McGill University's Faculty of Medicine to create a Department of Paediatrics until 1937, the same year the Canadian specialty board was created.[58] Although he was appointed to the faculty in 1902, pediatrics did not appear in his academic title until 1920.[59]

By contrast, Hôpital Ste-Justine, a children's hospital started by French-speaking philanthropist Justine Lacoste-Beaubien in 1907, was enthusiastically supported by the French-speaking medical schools from the beginning. As a result, its architectural form derived from several large-scale building campaigns, unlike the rather piecemeal development of the Children's Memorial Hospital. Following its equally modest beginnings in houses, the new H-shaped, three-hundred-bed Ste-Justine opened in April 1914; a six-floor north wing was added in 1921–22, including accommodation for private patients, electrotherapy, radiotherapy, isolation, dispensaries, a laundry, and heating furnaces; and in 1925–27, a new south wing (of eight stories) was constructed and a fifth floor added to the center block (Figure 2.28). One hundred and fifty rooms for nurses were added

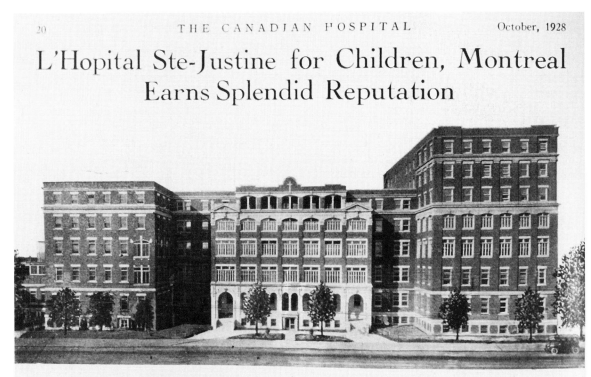

20   THE CANADIAN HOSPITAL   October, 1928

L'Hopital Ste-Justine for Children, Montreal Earns Splendid Reputation

A front view of the imposing Ste-Justine Hospital, Montreal

FIGURE 2.28. Hôpital Ste-Justine represented the ultimate in a scientific children's hospital.

then, too. In 1932, a nurses' home, labs, and laundry were added. All four buildings were designed by Montrealer Joseph Sawyer, architect of a number of hospitals such as the first general hospital for women in Canada, Montreal's Women's General Hospital (1927; its name was changed to the Herbert Reddy Memorial Hospital in 1946), and the Hôpital Notre-Dame de la Merci (1932), as well as schools, churches, and other important Catholic institutions.[60]

Hôpital Ste-Justine represented the ultimate in a scientific children's hospital; its design could not have differed more from the architecture of the Children's Memorial. Whereas the anglophone hospital presumed poor families would benefit from its lofty location, Ste-Justine was sited on north St. Denis Street, "where the population mainly comprises families of workmen."[61] And whereas the Children's Memorial Hospital was made up of a dozen or so small pavilions, terraced into the mountain, Ste-Justine was an integrated urban mass. The francophone hospital included all the features associated with the modern institution: operating rooms, X-ray department, laboratories, dietetics. It was categorized as Class A by the American College of Surgeons.[62]

The relationship of pediatrics to other specialties, especially obstetrics, was also more clearly demarcated at Ste-Justine than in the Children's Memorial Hospital. In the course of expansion in 1928, Ste-Justine added a maternity ward and crèche to the new north wing. The service continued throughout the 1930s, with forty beds, forty bassinets, and three doctors. The Children's Memorial opened a ward for infants in 1914, but obstetrics/gynecology remained the responsibility of the Royal Victoria, cemented by the construction of Stevens and Lee's Montreal Royal Victoria Maternity Hospital in 1925–26. By contrast, at Hôpital Notre-Dame, the general hospital associated with Ste-Justine, pregnant women were not admitted unless they had a life-threatening condition.[63]

Historic photographs of the Children's Memorial Hospital and Hôpital Ste-Justine give further insight into the differing personalities of the two institutions. Not surprisingly, official images of the Children's Memorial Hospital, like the hand-tinted postcard of 1912 (Figure 2.29) and Notman's photograph of the hospital in 1913, emphasize its romantic forms and domestic associations. The upward angle of the postcard image, for example, sets off the varied rooftop elements of the building—gable-end chimneys, dormers, curved oriel window, and expressed parapets—features we associate with domestic rather than institutional design. The angle also showcases the hospital's bay window and fine brick detailing. The Children's Memorial Hospital's small scale, too, is reinforced by the relatively informal postures of the nurses shown in the postcard. One even sits on the ground in her starched white uniform. The same sort of images can be seen in an extant photo album belonging to Rose Wilkinson, a nurse at the Children's Memorial Hospital, which is mostly filled with snapshots of staff members and patients (Figure 2.30). These are intimate images of groups huddled together, often smiling and touching, resembling family photographs. Photographs of Ste-Justine's patients, on the other hand, are typically more formal, emphasizing the hospital's scientific, institutional character.

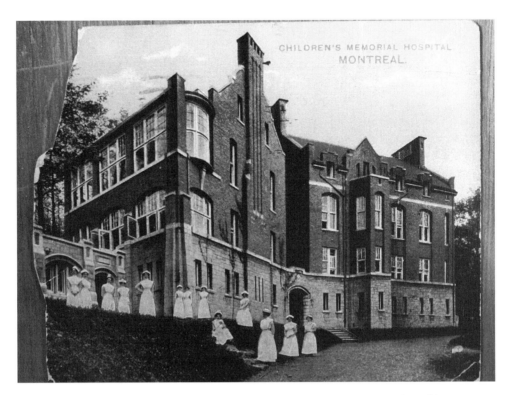

FIGURE 2.29. Images of the Children's Memorial Hospital emphasize its cozy, houselike aspects, circa 1912.

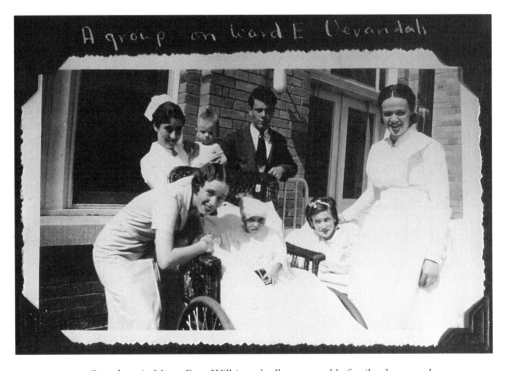

FIGURE 2.30. Snapshots in Nurse Rose Wilkinson's album resemble family photographs.

Comparing the design of Ste-Justine and the Children's Memorial Hospital also speaks eloquently of the differences between French and English children's hospitals in Montreal during the first half of the twentieth century. Perhaps most obviously, it should dispel the notion that francophone hospitals were somehow less scientific, or more backward, than their anglophone counterparts. This presumption was most clearly articulated by historian Shelley Hornstein, who suggested in a 1991 article on the architecture of Montreal's nineteenth-century teaching hospitals that the religious (French) and secular (English) institutions were in constant competition for the domination of Mount Royal. She sets the original Montreal General and the Hôtel-Dieu in opposition, describing the English system and its buildings as "an architecture of domination," while she reads the French hospital, mostly due to its convent-derived form, as a "zone of passivity." As further support for her thesis on the competitive nature of hospital building between Montreal's French- and English-speaking populations, Hornstein also reads the siting of these two buildings as a case of straightforward one-upmanship, remarking that nineteenth-century teaching hospitals in Montreal literally "leapfrog[ged] up its hills" in a competition "waged for the administration of life or the conquest of death."[64] The tensions that shaped twentieth-century children's hospitals, as should be clear by now, are more nuanced than their linguistic differences express.

In conclusion, even though children's hospitals and wards were fairly common in the interwar period, pediatrics had a difficult time establishing itself as a specialty. Separate facilities for young patients were evidence of their marginal status, unlike the situations of paying patients and pregnant women, whose separate facilities symbolized their high social standing. As we will see in chapter 3, separation was a key theme in the architecture designed for nurses and doctors, with social class and gender continuing to trump age, and scientific-looking spaces displacing domestic ideology as time progressed.

Nurses

3 THE ARCHITECTURE OF THE ROYAL VICTORIA HOSPITAL NURSES'
residence embodies two powerful ideological forces: the "bourgeois ideology of femininity," which attempted to "contain womens' work outside the home within the duties of homemaking," and the reformist
drive to professionalize nursing, which attempted to valorize women's
work inside the hospital by grounding it in theoretical and scientific
training.[1] While the building's eclectic ornament and domestic spaces
were intended to attract middle-class women to join the ranks of the
growing profession, these same architectural features simultaneously
limited women's participation in the world of health care to the same
roles they played in the middle-class family. Still, these buildings shaped
the Canadian nursing profession for the better, giving nurses control
of unmistakably identified space in which to live and work, in contrast
to their prior "invisible" occupation of the hospital. The residence's
clear connections to the hospital—both physical links and stylistic
congruities—acknowledged the students' grueling schedules and total
commitment to nursing. Precariously poised between public and private,
nurses' residences reveal the truly paradoxical relationship of domestic
and institutional architecture designed for women at this time. A real
"room of one's own," at least for nurses, offered both autonomy and
restraint at once.

THE NURSES' RESIDENCE

The numerous nurses' residences constructed during the first half of the twentieth century at many older hospitals were an important feature of the modernized institution. In Montreal, the Royal Victoria erected a residence in 1907, which received significant additions in 1917 and 1932; the Montreal General Hospital added a new residence in 1926; Hôpital Notre-Dame and Hôpital Ste-Justine, the French children's hospital discussed in chapter 2, followed in 1931. In eastern Ontario, the Kingston General Hospital's massive renovations, which began in 1916 "to make it modern in every respect," included a nurses' home by Stevens and Lee.[2] Perhaps the best example of a modern hospital built entirely by the firm, the Ottawa Civic Hospital included a freestanding home for 230 nurses in its initial design. Most significantly, all these buildings offered single women a place to live in the city, outside the traditional, middle-class home.

The desire for a homelike character may explain the choice of architects for the new nurses' residence at the Royal Victoria. In May 1905, McGill University professor Percy Nobbs recommended the design of Edward and William Sutherland Maxwell as the winner of a limited competition for the building.[3] The Maxwell brothers had designed many of the gracious mansions of the Square Mile, which hugged Mount Royal to the west of the hospital and was inhabited by the wealthy families who supported the hospital and attempted to direct its future. Other local architects were commissioned to extend the building soon after its completion. In 1917, Hutchison and Wood, who had placed second in the 1905 competition, designed an addition to the north of the Maxwells' building; the following year they added a kitchen (Figure 3.1). In 1931–32, the building was expanded once again. Lawson & Little's new wing to the west of the original nurses' home provided 132 additional rooms, as well as a gymnasium, a reference library, a dietetic laboratory, and lecture and demonstration rooms, for the escalating population of student nurses at the hospital (Figure 3.2).

The educational program for nurses based at the Royal Victoria Hospital did not begin with the realization of the new residence, designed by Edward and W. S. Maxwell in 1905. Since the founding of the Training School in October 1894, nursing students at the Royal Victoria Hospital had lived amidst the large, open wards, exposed to the fetid air, contagious diseases, and never-ending duties of turn-of-the-century nursing.[4] As domestic servants were expected to reside with the families who employed them, student nurses were required to live at the hospital, conforming to the rules and regulations of the institution.[5] At the nearby Montreal General Hospital, it was reported that nurses' sleeping quarters were infested with insects and rats.[6] In most general urban hospitals constructed before 1900, few of the women who worked day and night had rooms of their own.[7]

Snell's drawings for the hospital (used extensively in chapter 1) show the organization of these spaces intended for nurses in the original hospital. These drawings propose several conflicting planning suggestions for nurses' bedrooms, Training School headquarters,

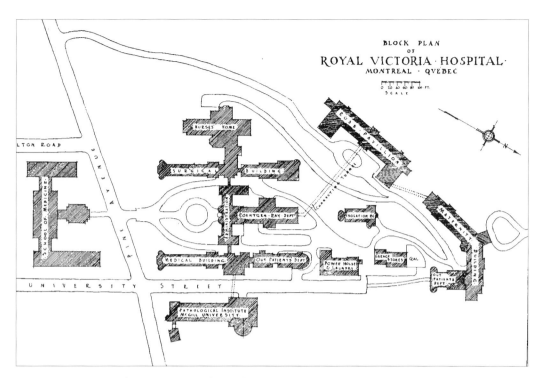

FIGURE 3.1. Royal Victoria Hospital, site plan.

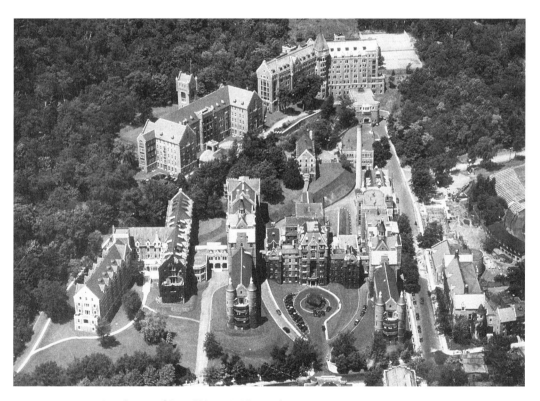

FIGURE 3.2. Aerial view of Royal Victoria Hospital, circa 1932.

and the Lady Superintendent's suite, spread over several floors in the main administration block. An early schematic axonometric block drawing of the complex, also drawn by Snell, places nurses in portions of central Blocks 7, 8, and 9, but subsequently the plans underwent many cuts and changes. Royal Vic historian David Sclater Lewis, however, explains authoritatively that on opening day "the Lady Superintendent's suite was situated on the second floor immediately over the front door of the hospital and her business office and the training School for Nurses occcupied similar space on the floor immediately above it. The nurses' quarters were on the fourth floor."[8] The rapid growth of the Training School soon put pressure on these accommodations, and the 1898 extension to the northeast end of the administration block, designed by Montreal architect Andrew Taylor, added a much-needed large dining room and bedrooms for nurses.[9] This dining room, illustrated in Lewis (Figure 10), was accessible from the hospital's main staircase.[10] Almost concurrently, in 1899, Taylor completed a five-story wing just north of the original Snell administration building to accommodate the congested outpatient department. It also included space for additional nurses' bedrooms on the fourth floor, visible in unsigned plans of the Royal Victoria dated May 13, 1905 (which were in the possession of the Maxwells). On the wards, where nurses could spend up to twenty-four hours a day, the original plans indicate only a tiny space for nurses "with inspecting windows, which command the entire wards."[11] Spaces for nurses, then, had no distinguishing architectural characteristics: no special entrances, circulation sequences, ornament, or massing.

The construction of the new residence was intended to improve the daily lives of the nurses at the busy urban hospital. Separate quarters were considered particularly imperative after a fire in 1905 damaged many of the nurses' bedrooms on the fourth floor of the Snell building, forcing them to sleep in the surgical wing for several months.[12] Adjoining the ventilation tower of Snell's surgical wing, the Maxwells' five-story, fireproof residence gave the nurses private space within their sphere of work and status and visibility in the community. In its heavy masonry construction, stepped gables, and details intended to evoke the institution's Scottish heritage, the new building mimicked, to some extent, its older neighbor, to which it was directly connected through a passageway above its east entrance.

Like the paying patients' pavilion would do a decade later, the Royal Victoria Hospital nurses' home drew heavily on middle-class domestic architecture, offering its aspiring residents 114 bedrooms, ten sitting rooms in which to socialize in small groups, a grand dining room, and a sequence of elegant spaces on its west side, including a library, living room, anteroom, and a large assembly hall with a stage (Figure 3.3). At the Ottawa Civic Hospital, too, Stevens and Lee's nurses' home featured a huge living room with a fireplace, located on axis with the main entrance and lobby. These spaces were deliberately homelike, intended to enact the residential function of the new buildings, and were given special emphasis in the massing of the buildings. A photo of the Ottawa Civic Hospital residence, for example, included in Stevens's book, shows how the large square living room protruded from the rectangular mass of the main residential section of the building. The living room windows were distinct from those of the bedrooms. The nurses' home as a building type, at the time of the Royal Victoria Hospital pavilion, was in the early stage of its development, long before the more institutional classrooms and demonstration labs characteristic of later nurses' homes.[13] By 1924, the opening date of the Ottawa Civic Hospital, these were included, beneath the living room on the basement level. In 1905, however, the education of nurses was still largely conducted in the hospital itself.[14]

The agitated silhouette of the home's stepped gables, which were presumably inspired by Snell's extensive use of the Scottish feature on the wards, ventilation towers, and administration block of the 1893 building (as discussed in chapter 1), added to its romanticism. So did the fact that it was the first major extension to the hospital to break the apparent symmetry of Snell's monumental courtyard. This bold gesture expressed

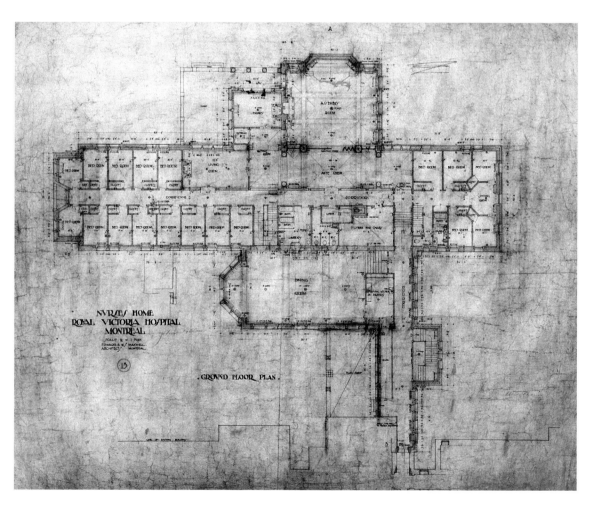

FIGURE 3.3. Ground floor plan of nurses' residence.

the newer building's noninstitutional nature, which was further differentiated by the proliferation of dormers and stone railings on the Maxwell building. Indeed, the Maxwells' own perspective view (Figure 3.4) emphasizes their building's isolation from the Snell hospital, whose west tower and ward loom behind the new building in the watercolor drawing. The vantage point selected for the rendering and for many photographs (Figure 3.5) of the building completely obscured the residence's physical connection to the hospital, making it appear, instead, as a freestanding, isolated (and therefore smaller, domestic) structure. Even the siting of the building at the Royal Victoria Hospital was romantic. Nestled among the trees and poised on the steep ground west of the Snell building, the original nurses' residence was only partially visible from Pine Avenue, the busy thoroughfare in front of the hospital. The winding pathways and obliquely placed gateways of the growing hospital complex ensured that the residence was mostly seen in oblique views (Figure 3.6).

This idea of a separate, seemingly domestic structure situated in a romantic landscape was essential to the experience of this first nurses' residence. In addition to the winding flagstone path, which one 1933 resident wrote "entices us to follow whither it doth lead; we yield and follow it to the door of the Home,"[15] the location of the nurses' residence to the west of the hospital ensured that it was seen against the backdrop of Mount Royal's wooded slopes. The area above the original hospital was vacant at this time; Nobbs's own Pathological Institute was constructed to the east in 1924, across University Street from the Snell building.

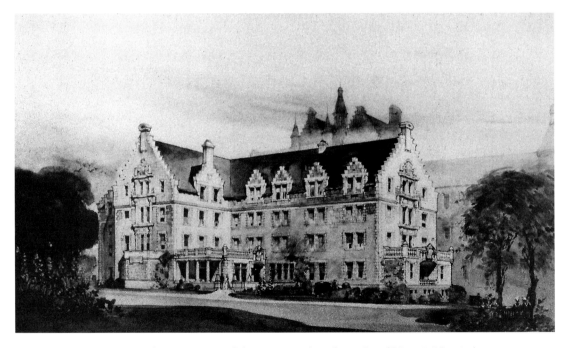

FIGURE 3.4. Watercolor perspective of the new nurses' residence, Royal Victoria Hospital.

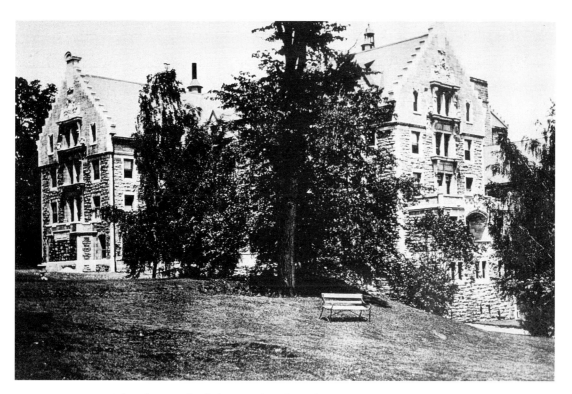

FIGURE 3.5. This photograph of the nurses' residence from 1907 hides the huge hospital to which it is connected.

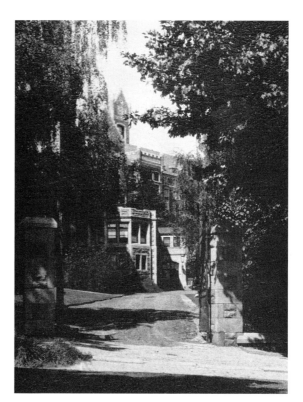

FIGURE 3.6. Entry and gate to the nurses' residence, Royal Victoria Hospital, 1917.

As was the case with many late-nineteenth-century institutions for women, particularly colleges, it is likely that the western site was considered more appropriate for the nurses' residence because of its more natural, untouched character. This association of women and nature was central to the process of suburbanization in the nineteenth century, as well as in the location of the first colleges for women at universities, which were typically relegated to the periphery of the campuses or even cities. It stemmed from long-established conceptions of nature, understood in the late nineteenth century as healthier, safer, and more beautiful than the unpredictable, industrialized city.[16] In the cases of both suburbs and early colleges, this widespread belief that women required protection from the dangers of urban life meant that they were removed or separated from centers of power, which tended to be located in more urban (less natural) locations.[17]

For a century, the eastern section of the large Royal Victoria Hospital site (both sides of University Street) has arguably been used as a more masculine, technology-oriented (urban) area. In addition to several prestigious medical buildings, it housed the power house/laundry building (1900) and ambulance garages (1911).[18] The western and northern edge of the roughly triangular site—the steep, rocky, wooded mountainside—was reserved for women (and wealthier patients).[19] This edge still today is marked by the Allan Memorial (a renovated mansion), the former nurses' residence, the Ross Memorial Pavilion (1915–16), and the maternity hospital (1925–26). Just beyond lie the heavily wooded, rocky slopes of Mount Royal.

Despite the separateness of the building as expressed in the drawing and photos, the actual connection of the nurses' residence to the hospital building proper was a blatant statement of the institution's expectation of total commitment on the part of its student nurses. The narrow passage, carefully detailed by the architects, expressed—maybe even ensured—the fact that the nurses' six-and-a-half-day work week left little time for any life outside the hospital.[20] The actual intersection of the hospital and nurses' residence was given elaborate architectural attention; the Maxwells designed a special door for the juncture.[21] Its decorative ironwork must have warned unwelcome visitors of the more private, domestic quarters beyond.

This close connection between hospital and nurses' residence was uncharacteristic of buildings constructed later in the century. Indeed, the influential *Survey of Nursing Education in Canada*, conducted by George Weir in 1932, recommended that nurses' residences be separated from hospitals, allowing "adequate opportunity for privacy, rest, quiet and retirement for study and for cultural recreation."[22] By then the modernization of both the hospital and the profession of nursing (and, indeed, the social advancement of women in general) meant that nurses could demand a certain degree of autonomy from the hospital. This autonomy was expressed in spatial terms by the physical distance separating their places of residence and work. Edward Stevens described the separation of residence and hospital in the 1920s as beneficial to the patients, taking the nurses' need for recreation for granted:

Any hospital of considerable size should have its nurses' residence. This should be a separate building, not too remote from the hospital, but far enough away so that the noises of an entertainment, a dancing party or a romp will not disturb the patients.[23]

Stevens also emphasized the need for nurses to "go out of the environment of the sick room, out of the sound of suffering, out of hospital smells, and in fact out of the hospital atmosphere."[24] In this earlier period of development, however, the need for nurses to escape their workplace was unacknowledged in spatial terms.

Domestic Interiors

The building's interiors, too, looked residential in terms of their physical form, as well as their intended use. Photographs of the new wing added by Lawson & Little in 1931–32 show the social spaces typically provided for nurses throughout the century. The new reference library, for example, replaced the earlier library by the Maxwells, which was subsumed in the new wing's entrance, while a new gymnasium extended from the Maxwells' original reception room (Figure 3.7).[25] These rooms were furnished with

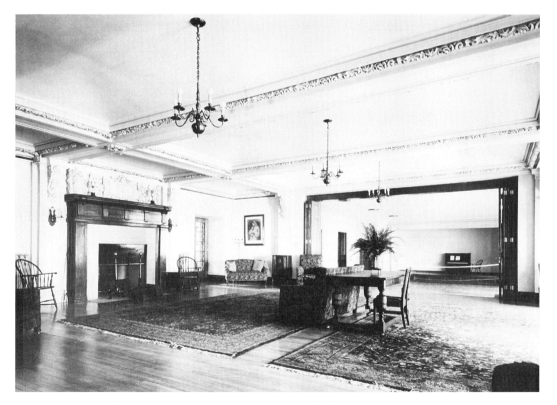

FIGURE 3.7. This gymnasium-reception room was typical of the multipurpose spaces included in early-twentieth-century nurses' residences.

comfortable, mass-produced chairs and tables, typical of middle-class houses at the time. The furniture was arranged casually, loosely grouped around fireplaces and pianos, probably intended to simulate intimate, homelike gatherings.

The nurses' yearbook praises the domestic character of the new residence, remarking on the foyer's "soft lights," which, one author suggested, "invite us to linger." The reception room on the first floor, "tastefully and comfortably furnished," was the setting for bridge parties and teas, rituals associated with middle-class women's lives that took place at home. The library, also illustrated in the yearbook, was "luxuriously furnished with piano, chesterfields and occasional chairs."[26]

Although there were no special apartment buildings for working women constructed in Montreal, as there were in both New York and London, the city had a well-established landscape of residences for women.[27] Montreal's many convents constitute an interesting example of extremely sophisticated (and large) residential blocks, which were often combined with enormous hospitals.[28] Like the Royal Victoria Hospital, the convents were typically H- or U-shaped ensembles of narrow greystone buildings. The Montreal convent was usually four or five stories, capped by steep gable or hipped roofs with dormer windows. Convent elevations featured repetitive rows of uniform windows, with little indication of the variety of complex, overlapping functions within the building. These included schools, orphanages, hospitals, massive kitchens, chapels, industrial spaces, and bedrooms for nuns.

A closer neighbor to the Royal Victoria Hospital was the Royal Victoria College. The first residential college for women at McGill University, it was founded in 1896.[29] The original Royal Victoria College building, designed by the well-known American architect Bruce Price, was completed in 1899.[30] It had classrooms and a huge dining room on the ground floor, while the assembly hall, library, parlor, and more classrooms were on the first story. The upper two floors of the Royal Victoria College had variously shaped bedrooms and shared sitting rooms, arranged along a straight corridor. The hospital and the residential college shared more than names and a concern for women; both were established through bequests by wealthy benefactor Donald A. Smith, Lord Strathcona, discussed in chapter 1. Not surprisingly, it was he who approved the idea of a separate building as a home for nurses at the Royal Victoria Hospital.[31]

Martha Vicinus has pointed out how many early buildings for women—colleges, schools, settlement houses—looked like large houses. This domestic imagery was probably intended to smooth the transition for middle-class women to the world of paid work, while at the same time offering the promise of gentle protection in that realm. "The surroundings," says Vicinus of the first colleges for women in England, "bespoke permanence, seriousness of purpose, and the same solidity that marked the middle-class families from which the bulk of them came."[32] The houselike appearance of the Royal Victoria Hospital nurses' residence probably assured anxious parents, too, that their daughters would be looked after, protected, and separated from the hospital, the street, and the city beyond.

Nursing professionals may also have presumed that the association of the residence with upper-middle-class houses would attract young women from wealthier (at least middle-class) families. In turn, the presence of nurses from wealthier families was one of the ways hospitals were made appealing to middle-class families after World War I. Just as the crisp, white nurses' uniforms made young graduates feel "dignified and poised," the new building may have imposed middle-class values on working-class women, whose backgrounds were increasingly unacceptable to the profession in the decades following Florence Nightingale's sweeping reforms.[33] Architects worked explicitly with these presumptions. Stevens pointed to the domestic character of the architecture, underlining its potential to attract wealthier nurses and to improve their performance, benefiting patients, too:

> The more attractive and homelike this building can be made and the more alluring it can be made to the young woman who is taking up nursing, the better will be the class of women who will come to it and, in the end, the better will be the care that the patient will receive.[34]

From this perspective, Nobbs had chosen the ideal architects as winners of the limited competition; the Maxwells were masters of domestic design. Indeed, mansions designed by the brothers in the surrounding neighborhood for prominent officers and benefactors of the hospital featured many of the same characteristics as the nurses' residence. Henry Vincent Meredith was president of the Royal Victoria Hospital from 1913 to 1929. His family's home, built in 1894, was probably the closest Maxwell house in terms of physical proximity to the hospital. It comprised elegant public rooms, expressed on the building's exterior, with private family spaces (Figure 3.8).[35] Like the nurses' residence, it boasted fine wood paneling and gracious circulation sequences; like all upper-middle-class residences of its time, it saw the strict separation of family and servants, men and women, adults and children. Its rooms were highly specialized and elaborately decorated. It is thus not surprising that this house (and several others designed by the Maxwells) became part of the institution when bequeathed to the hospital later in the century.[36]

Multifunctional Spaces

In spite of the traditional, domestic attributes of the nurses' residence, the building type became a trademark feature of the "modern" hospital throughout urban North America. An implicit assumption in the development of the type was that the more efficient the nurses' residence, the more efficient the hospital in general. This led to the gradual inclusion of educational spaces within the program of the nurses' home, a mark of both decreasing reliance on the hospital per se as the primary site of nursing education, and of increased specialization within the nursing profession. "Modern" nurses' residences built after 1920 included multifunctional social spaces, able to accommodate complex changes in use, relative to the earlier near-imitation of traditional domestic spaces. An example of this is the transformation of the Maxwells' assembly room of 1905 into the expanded assembly room/gymnasium space of Lawson & Little in the 1930s. "It is a convertible room appearing now as a ballroom, now a gymnasium and again as a lecture theatre, seating comfortably two hundred and fifty persons," boasted the *1933 Yearbook.* Despite this "modern," multifunctional conception of the room, social rooms in nurses' residences were typically furnished in an extremely traditional manner. The rooms at the Royal Victoria Hospital, for example, featured oriental rugs, upholstered armchairs and couches, Windsor chairs, and heavy draperies with sheers. Their modernism, that is, was wholly derived from their use, not their look. As we will see in chapter 5, this ploy of disguising new types of hospital spaces in traditionalist or historicist imagery is a recurring theme in the modern hospital.

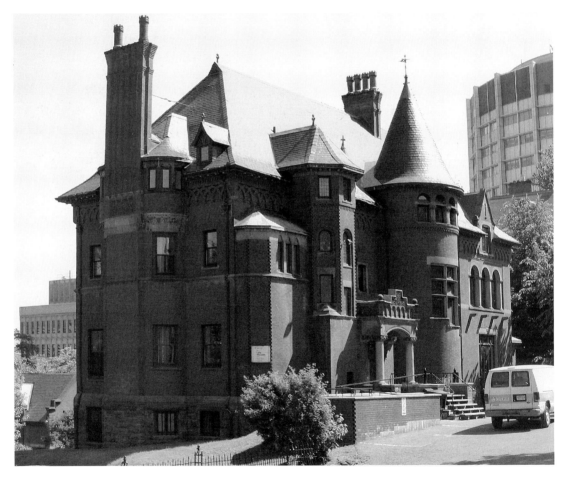

FIGURE 3.8. The Meredith house was designed by the same firm as the nurses' residence and featured similar planning ideas.

By this time educational spaces were fully integrated into nurses' residences. The basement level had ample areas dedicated to classrooms and laboratories (Figure 3.9).[37] Although this teaching unit occupied an entire floor, these rooms received no special treatment in the massing or elevations of the extension. In terms of planning, however, the educational rooms were considered extremely up-to-date, organized as they were on "scientific" principles. The classroom, for example, had a sloping floor, allowing each nursing student to view the blackboard in the front of the room; the demonstration room included beds, model trays, and mannequins, simulating the real hospital environment next door, but under more regulated circumstances.[38]

This notion of control pervaded the architectural design. At the same time as the building saw the introduction of these supposedly modern features, the nurses' residence remained an arena in which the hospital administration could closely supervise and control the private lives of nursing professionals. Student nurses could not marry; they kept strict curfews and their friendships were carefully monitored.[39] In the 1920s, nurses were required to wear hats when leaving the building and to return home by 10:00 p.m. Smoking, dating the so-called housemen (the British term for resident and intern physicians), or mentioning the issue of salary were strictly prohibited.[40]

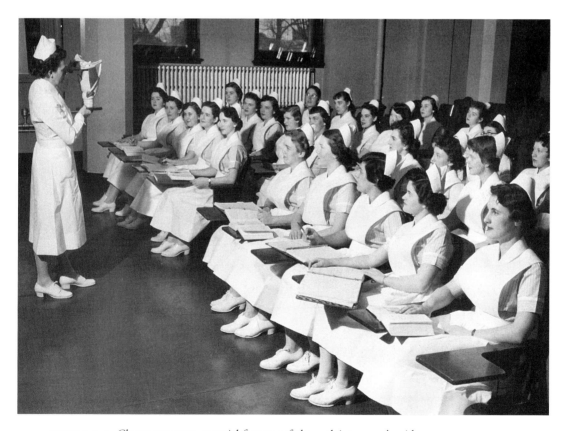

FIGURE 3.9. Classrooms were essential features of the evolving nurses' residence.

Lawson & Little's monumental extension to the Maxwells' building in the early 1930s gave physical form to many of these restrictions imposed on nurses' lives. The new building continued the general massing of the earlier residence, extending the west end of the Maxwell project with a new entry sequence (through the former Maxwell library). This hallway led to the generous gymnasium behind the former stage of the Maxwell assembly room. A medieval-revival tower housed the elevator, another modern feature cloaked in traditional imagery. The tower marked the crossing of this long hallway and the double-loaded corridor that commanded the more residential section of the new extension. Like the educational rooms in the basement, bedrooms in the new wing were considered completely up-to-date, "artistically furnished in a green, rose or tangerine colour scheme."[41] The section of the building running from the elevator lobby in the tower southward toward Pine Avenue was even known as "peacock alley," because of its bright colors, highly decorated appearance, and the omnipresence of nursing supervisors.[42] Special bedroom furniture, like the multifunctional social spaces in the new wing, served several purposes at once. A single piece functioned as dresser, desk, and bookcase, for example.[43]

SPATIAL CONFINEMENT

The expansion of the residence so soon after its completion may have sprung from the hospital's desire to segregate nurses even more than the 1905 building had prescribed. Of great concern to the hospital administration, after all, was that even after the construction of the original residence, student nurses continued to have close contact with the male staff. In the early 1920s, for example, when the Maxwell building could no longer accommodate the total number of nurses working at the Royal Victoria Hospital, students whose names began with the letters A through J were housed in part of the former Ward K, which had been converted into a temporary residence. The other half of the former ward was occupied by the interns, separated from the student nurses by only a particle board partition. "In no time a direct communication system had been established," recounted Eileen Flanagan fifty years later, "by means of a clothesline stretched across the alleyway between the two wings. Many a note and batches of homemade candy were passed across."[44]

This notion of the necessary spatial confinement of nurses was expressed in the Canadian architectural press throughout the twentieth century. Advertisements for building products in the *Journal of the Royal Architectural Institute of Canada*, for example, into the 1960s, frequently featured nurses with architectural components that emphasized hygiene, safety, and quiet (Figure 3.10).[45] Nurses shown with locks and doors emphasized their roles as guardians of the all-important threshold. This pointed juxtaposition with doors and door hardware may also have been a symbolic reference to nurses' purity and chastity; the thresholds depicted in the press, in this way, implied the containment of women in hospital settings largely controlled by men.

SILENT DOORS
without this ⟶

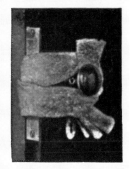

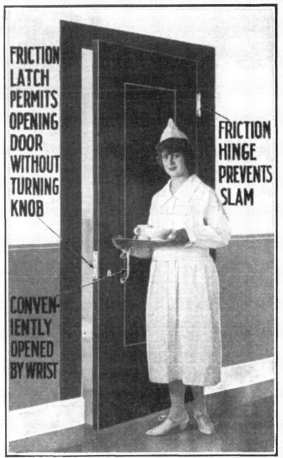

FRICTION LATCH PERMITS OPENING DOOR WITHOUT TURNING KNOB

FRICTION HINGE PREVENTS SLAM

CONVEN-IENTLY OPENED BY WRIST

You can open doors conveniently *with your elbows* —you can open them silently and without clicking the latches when you use the beautiful Rayco Hospital Hardware. And, with Rayco Friction Hinges, you can let doors swing closed without slamming!

Sanitary, durable, practical and handsome Rayco Hospital Hardware is used wherever smartness and silence is desired.

Complete information gladly sent by

RAYMER HARDWARE CO.

2373 University Ave.
St. Paul, Minn.

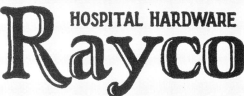

HOSPITAL HARDWARE
Rayco

Inquire about the New RAYCO Card Holder

FIGURE 3.10. Nurses were frequently featured in advertisements of door locks.

Nurses at the Royal Victoria Hospital were constantly threatened with expulsion and "never made to feel that we were in any way indispensable to the illustrious establishment." "Well, it will only take a car ticket to take you home," claimed Lady Superintendent of Nurses Mabel Hersey to Flanagan in 1920, when she was a new student. Nellie Goodhue, a teacher who herself had been a member of the first graduating class, repeatedly told her probationers: "If any of you wishes to leave, it will cause no more effect than dipping a finger in a pail of water and pulling it out."[46]

The confinement, surveillance, and discipline of student nurses in early-twentieth-century hospitals were primarily the responsibility of the head nurse, or Lady Superintendent. Most drastically, Lady Superintendents exercised their power by threatening the dismissal of resident student nurses who broke the regulations. Lawson & Little's plans of the early 1930s reflect the important place occupied by Hersey, who was superintendent from 1908 to 1938 and figured centrally in the development of nursing education and the profession in Quebec.[47] While the inclusion of the classrooms, library, and gymnasium must have appeared as fairly progressive at the time—the institution's maintenance of the students' minds and bodies—the subtle renovations made to the Maxwell building by the later architects are extremely telling. Four bedrooms in the south end of the original building were transformed at the time of the new addition into a relatively luxurious four-room apartment for Hersey. Critical to its function in the growing complex, of course, was the new suite's strategic position overlooking the entrance area and stairs. Inside the building, Hersey could easily survey peacock alley, the long corridor of the residence's main floor.

This form of direct surveillance was unknown in other residential sections of the hospital complex. It may not have even occurred in the earlier separate nurses' residence constructed in 1905: the Medical Board had suggested that the Lady Superintendent's quarters should remain in the administration building, and the Maxwells' floor plans have no textual or graphic indications of a special suite for the Lady Superintendent.[48] For example, the first male superintendent, who was in charge of the entire hospital, did not live at the hospital, underlining again this important question of which employees were permitted to live apart from their place of work.[49]

THE INTERNS' RESIDENCE

In direct contrast to the situation of nurses, medical interns, the housemen who also lived at the hospital, moved freely throughout the institution and were seen as fundamental members of the hospital establishment. In 1930, the Royal Victoria Hospital constructed a special residence for interns, designed by Ross & Macdonald, on the foundation of Ward S, the old isolation pavilion and original hospital laundry building. The new four-story, fireproof home for forty interns was located directly behind Snell's administration block, in a commanding position at the center of the entire complex, between the historic building and the new, more "scientific" hospitals designed by Stevens and Lee, which had been constructed up the hill (discussed in chapter 2).[50] Like the nurses' residence, the interns' building was a long, narrow structure with stepped gables at its ends (Figure 3.11).

Social spaces provided for the interns were intended to encourage qualities associated with masculinity and power; the first-floor billiards room (Figure 3.12) was featured prominently in photographs of the hospital's resident interns.[51] Billiards was a popular game played by aristocratic men at home or at businesss clubs, and it was associated with drinking, smoking, and gambling. Billiards rooms were common in luxurious houses, often adjacent to the dining room (a masculine room) or in the basement. The interns' residence billiards table makes a neat comparison to the piano, a standard feature of nurses' residences. Whereas billiards is a competitive game that tests individual dexterity and the intern's ability to strategize, playing the piano showcases a nurse's artistic talent and ability to communicate emotional sensitivity. On the one hand, as a piece of furniture the piano brought nurses together to sing or just listen. For interns, on the other

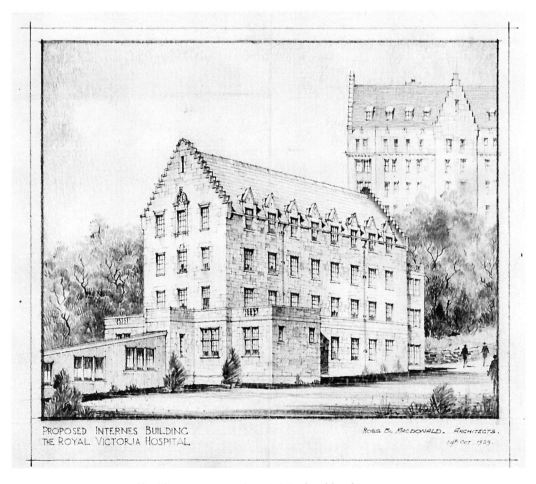

PROPOSED INTERNES BUILDING
THE ROYAL VICTORIA HOSPITAL

ROSS & MACDONALD. ARCHITECTS.
14ᵗ OCT 1929.

FIGURE 3.11. Interns' building perspective, Ross & Macdonald architects, 1929.

hand, the billiard table may have offered a solitary escape. Its referents are business, politics, and gambling; the piano recalled churches and family life.

Promotional photographs showing a typical day in the life of an intern featured him in active modes, often controlling new technology or performing medical procedures. Interns were men of science, who analyzed X-rays, peered into microscopes, kept up-to-date in somber libraries, and cured patients on the spot. Nurses, in contrast, were more typically pictured in groups and nearly always at rest. Featured in the hospital's promotional material gathered around a piano, engaging in informal conversations, or watching television, nurses were at home in the hospital. In the enormous complex of the modern hospital, doctors in training were pictured as men at work; student nurses, as women of leisure. The planning of the hospital is material evidence of these starkly different roles for male and female health-care providers trained in the modern hospital.

Today, the section of the Royal Victoria Hospital that once housed its student nurses is generally indistinguishable from the rest of the institution. Its finely crafted interiors have given way to the more anonymous, undecorated, "scientific" design of postwar hospital architecture. The only traces of its tenure as purpose-built architecture for women are in extant architectural drawings and photographs, preserved largely because the original building and its additions were designed by relatively well-known architects. The mere footprint of the nurses' residences in the ensemble, nonetheless, is a potent reminder of women's struggle for visibility and autonomy in the modern hospital.

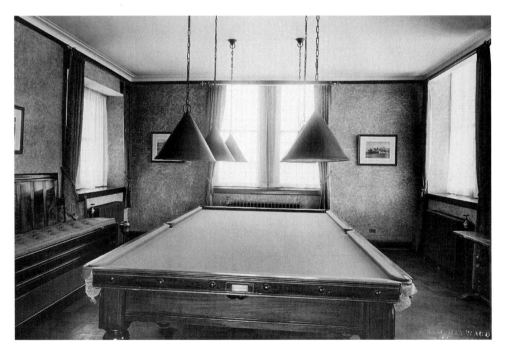

FIGURE 3.12. Doctors in training played billiards, a sharp contrast to the gathering of nurses around the piano.

Architects
and Doctors

4

THE PRECEDING CHAPTERS HAVE TAKEN US ON SELECTED TOURS OF the hospital, from the drafty, open wards of the sprawling pavilion-plan hospital of 1893 to the luxurious private patients' quarters of 1930. Along the way, we have stopped to appreciate why children's and women's hospitals are both separate from the main hospital (yet in different ways and for different reasons); why nurses' residences look like houses; and what a billiards table says about medical education, among other places and questions. Chapter 5 will synthesize some architectural features and ideas our detailed tour missed, summing up the changes in design the hospital endured from 1893 to 1943 and explaining the apparent contradiction between historicist imagery and modern design.

Behind many of these design reforms hovers the figure of the specialized hospital architect, a phenomenon introduced in chapter 1. This chapter argues that in the early years of the twentieth century, the responsibility for design shifted with the appearance of a burgeoning constellation of hospital experts and the fracturing of the hospital into constituent parts. A second intention here is to show how the tensions between architects and doctors shaped design decisions. Disagreements over the appropriateness of natural lighting in the surgical suite, for example, illustrate such a conflict in expertise.

Twentieth-century architects' approach to hospital design differed substantially from the generation of Henry Saxon Snell. As we saw in chapter 1, Snell produced huge, pavilion-plan hospitals across the British Empire. He conceptualized each pavilion-plan hospital he designed holistically. To Snell, the image of the hospital and its function were inextricably linked. He and his firm, including his sons, were responsible for every aspect of their design, from the overall site plan to the ventilating tubes. Snell's career and reputation were built on the similitaries of the hospital to related building types, such as poor houses and orphanages. Specialist architects in North America whose careers peaked in the post–World War I era defined their expertise not so much in the hospital's linkage to other reform institutions as in its close connection to the practice of medicine. The plan of the hospital, in particular, and its relationship to medicine became especially important. Sir Henry C. Burdett, author of *Hospitals and Asylums of the World* (1891) and Snell's contemporary, commented on this change in 1916:

> The esthetic features of the new building may not be overlooked, but the arrangement of the rooms (the making of the plan) is fundamental and of the greater importance. A lack of realization of this fact, and an incomplete knowledge of the real needs and purposes of the hospital on the part of the building committee, are the greatest difficulties usually encountered by the hospital adviser, architect, engineer and builder.[1]

Like Burdett, architect Edward F. Stevens identified the "making of the plan" as the substance of his own dominant position in the field of hospital design. As we will see in chapter 5, Stevens saw the plan of the building and the design of its exterior as separate domains, even inferring that only the plan of the hospital might require his expertise. This new, relatively exclusive focus on planning was a defining characteristic of early-twentieth-century hospital expertise.

Stevens's Career

Stevens, his longtime partner Frederick Lee, and several members of their office staff were on the forefront of this change. Stevens, in particular, exemplifies this significant transformation in the dynamics of hospital expertise from the late nineteenth to the early twentieth century, especially in his rather unique role as a nonmedically trained expert and author. Born October 2, 1860, in Dunstable, Massachusetts, Stevens (Figure 4.1) enrolled at the Massachusetts Institute of Technology as a special student in architecture for the second term of the academic year 1881–82 and the first and second terms of the year 1882–83.[2] He subsequently worked as a draftsman for Allen & Kenway and then for McKim, Mead & White as clerk of the works on the Boston Public Library.[3] In 1890, he formed a partnership with Henry H. Kendall in Boston, under the name of Kendall & Stevens. During 1896–97, the firm was sometimes known as Rand & Taylor, Kendall & Stevens. The seeds of Stevens's burgeoning career as a hospital specialist, however, were sown sometime about 1898. From 1898 to 1907, as a partner in the Boston-based firm of Kendall, Taylor, and Stevens, the architect designed a number of significant hospitals in New England.[4]

HOUSES AND HOSPITALS

Stevens's early experience was mostly in the design of large private houses, rather than benevolent public institutions. Kendall & Stevens designed a number of large dwellings in the northeastern United States, several of which were published in major architectural journals. For example, the house for Mrs J. H. Burleigh, in South Berwick, Maine, appeared in *The American Architect and Building News.* The architects' perspective (Figure 4.2) shows a monumental, Colonial Revival house, featuring a gallery, porte cochere, two round towers, Corinthian-style columns (doubled on the gallery), dormer windows with alternating pediment designs, and a widow's walk framed by massive chimneys. Interiors designed by the firm included classical details, too. The Green house at Jamaica Plain (Mass.) of 1896, designed by Rand & Taylor, Kendall & Stevens, featured a living room (Figure 4.3) with a coffered ceiling, wall niches for classical statues, paneled, built-in seating, and a square, fluted column.

The use of domestic imagery in hospitals was common during Stevens's early career. It wasn't unusual for hospitals to be converted houses, and many purpose-built hospitals drew on residential prototypes. *The American Architect* published only a partial elevation and wall section of the administration building of the Faulkner Hospital in West Roxbury,

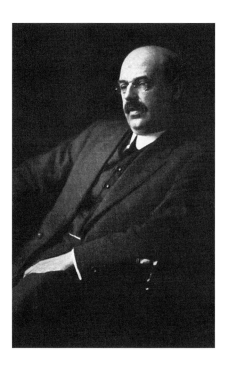

FIGURE 4.1. Portrait of hospital architect Edward Fletcher Stevens.

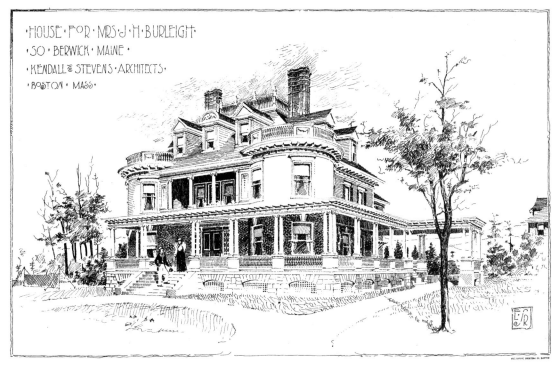

FIGURE 4.2. Stevens's early career was devoted to domestic design, such as the Burleigh house by Kendall & Stevens, South Berwick, Maine.

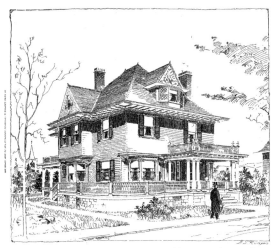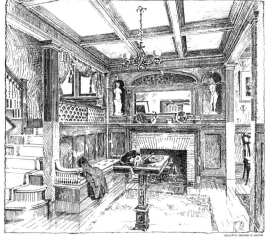

FIGURE 4.3. The Green house by Rand & Taylor and Kendall & Stevens, Jamaica Plain, Massachusetts, featured elegant interiors.

Massachusetts, in 1902. These drawings show the rather elaborate brick and terra cotta details of the building. Like the Burleigh house, the Faulkner hospital had a cast-iron widow's walk and dormer windows with rather exquisite decoration. The building for acute patients at the Massachusetts Hospital for the Insane in Westborough (Figure 4.4), among the earliest hospitals published by the firm, included spatial elements of domestic design. The two-story building featured a two-story porch-balcony with a classical railing and a steep hipped roof with dormers. Only the plan, which included turkish baths, two solaria, generous dayrooms and wards, and separate entrances for men and women, hinted at the institutional mandate of the building.

The link between houses and hospitals was important to Stevens throughout his career, even long after he stopped designing residential architecture. In 1918, he wrote a prominent article, published in both the medical and architectural presses, explaining how to turn a house into a hospital, perhaps recalling his early days of designing hospitals that resembled large houses (and Roman temples).[5] And in many projects he consciously modeled the hospital on domestic architecture.

Although Kendall, Taylor & Stevens's work is closely linked to the domestic design of the late nineteenth century, the firm was clearly aware of hospital architecture, too.

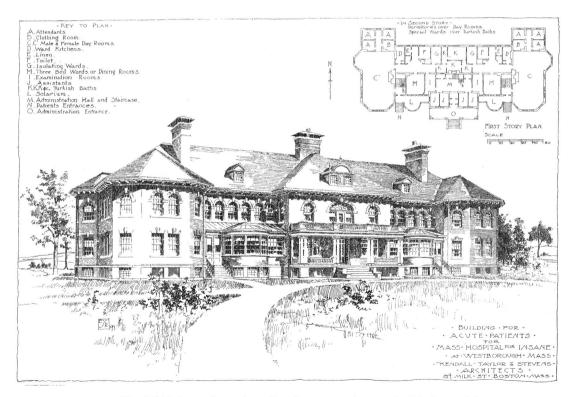

FIGURE 4.4. Kendall, Taylor & Stevens's pavilion for acute patients at the Westborough Insane Hospital, Massachusetts, is an example of a houselike institution.

The Beverly Hospital (Figure 4.5), in Beverly, Massachusetts, illustrates the persistence of the pavilion plan. The plan called for two double-story rectangular pavilions (each ward included ten beds), connected to a Roman Revival administration building with open corridors. A fourth building designed for surgery, to the southeast of one of the pavilions, broke the symmetry of the rather old-fashioned (by this date) organization.

The Architect as Traveler and Writer

Relatively little is known about Stevens's work during the first decade of the twentieth century. In 1911, he embarked on a European tour that affirmed his hospital knowledge, traveling to Amsterdam, The Hague, Utrecht, Hamburg, Berlin, Dresden, Vienna, Paris, and London with Dr. John Nelson Elliot Brown, superintendent of the Toronto General Hospital from 1905 to 1911.[6] Stevens had also traveled to Europe in 1907 (he practiced independently from 1907 to 1912), at which time he visited the Pasteur Institute in Paris, an institution that influenced his work in North America.[7] Travel provided the opportunity not only to see significant models but also to photograph them. During the 1911 trip, Stevens collected images of buildings, which he used throughout his career in presentations to hospital boards.

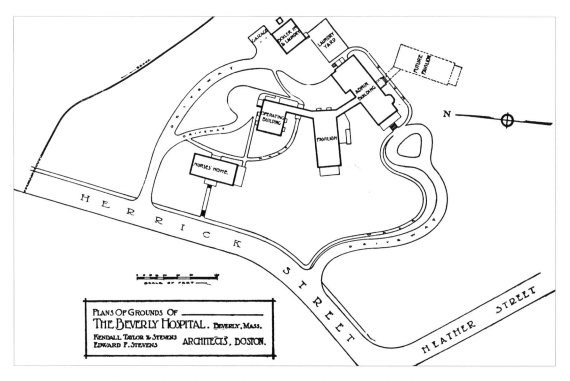

FIGURE 4.5. The site plan of Kendall, Taylor & Stevens's Beverly Hospital shows the persistence of the pavilion plan typology.

Stevens's visits to hospitals abroad sharpened his personal knowledge of various issues in hospital design. And, he used his newfound knowledge and photos in his publishing ventures. He and Brown coauthored a chapter in Charlotte Aikens's *Hospital Management,* the same year that they traveled together to Europe, as well as an article about the trip in *Hospital World.*[8] The chapter in *Hospital Management* foretold the outline of Stevens's 1918 book in terms of its general organization. Perhaps the most interesting aspect of the coauthored venture, however, was the presentation of an ideal one-hundred-bed hospital that comprised separate buildings (connected underground) on a rural site. Their plan of the Infectious building, in particular, showed the direct influence of the Pasteur Institute, in that the entire wall separating the rooms from the corridor was glass and that visitors were limited to a continuous balcony that ran the length of the building. The 1911 European tour was also the basis of his lifelong interest in hydrotherapy, an unorthodox medical treatment involving the use of water to treat pains and diseases.[9] The basic idea of hydroptherapy in Stevens's era was to transfer heat and cold by means of general and local baths.

Stevens's work also appeared in important books written or edited by others. His article on the details and equipment of hospitals was included in the book *Modern Hospital,* which summarized material he had first delivered at the 1911 American Hospital Association meeting in New York. The other authors included an architect, two engineers, and a hospital superintendent from Manila. Like his own book seven years later, this article included many photographs and references to the hospitals he had seen on his European tours in 1907 and 1911, particularly the St. Georg Hospital at Hamburg. In the conclusion of the article, in fact, Stevens claims to have visited more than thirty-five hospitals in Europe.

Stevens's development as North America's top hospital architect ran parallel to the rise of specialized hospital magazines, like *Modern Hospital* (begun in 1913) and *Canadian Hospital* (begun in 1924), which were crucial to the dissemination of his work. Typically, hospital journals ran extensive, generously illustrated articles on new facilities, including lengthy accounts of their site planning, layout, and details. Descriptions of the projects may have been sent out from the hospitals or offices like Stevens's, since there are many repetitions among the articles, and there is never any critical commentary on the projects. Nearly all these articles included the plans of the hospitals, Stevens's hallmark.[10]

Although the inclusion of his projects in journals was clearly important to the firm, *The American Hospital of the Twentieth Century* remained Stevens's most significant publication, appearing in three editions (1918, 1921, 1928). With each subsequent publication of the book, Stevens included more and more of his own work. The revised edition of 1921 included 150 new illustrations; the 1928 edition presented a full array of Stevens and Lee projects completed in the decade since the book first appeared, including both pavilions at the Royal Victoria Hospital, the Ottawa Civic, and Hôpital Notre-Dame. This final edition of *The American Hospital of the Twentieth Century* resulted from "the fact that first and second editions of this book have been exhausted." Stevens also emphasized in the new foreword to this edition that the period since 1923 had "shown a more marked development in hospital planning than any previous twenty years," perhaps reflecting upon his own busy practice at this time. Not coincidentally, the book was organized along the lines of the hospital—by department. Stevens devoted entire chapters to the ward unit, surgical unit, medical unit, maternity department, children's hospital, as well as contagious, psychopathic, and tuberculosis departments. The second half of the book is dedicated to special departments, small hospitals, the housing of nurses, mechanical services, construction, equipment, and hospital landscapes.

The book was closely tied to the architect's travels. A reviewer of the original edition in 1918 summed up Stevens's intersecting interests in the journal *Hospital World:* "The author has travelled much, observing closely, noting carefully and reproducing faithfully."[11]

Following the third and final edition of the book in 1928, the firm's structure and clientele changed. In 1933, it became Stevens, Curtin, & Mason; by 1941, it was Stevens, Curtin, Mason & Riley.[12] With the changing partnerships came new international commissions. Among Stevens's last projects were the Mixto and Maternidad hospitals in Lima, Peru. He retired in 1943, on the brink of an entirely new era in hospital architecture.

Stevens's book was one among a handful of popular books on hospital design, written by architects, available in the interwar era. A 1929 article described Charles Butler and Stevens as "outstanding architects in hospital work."[13] Butler's book *Hospital Planning* followed an outline remarkably similar to Stevens's. He included several of Stevens's hospitals in *Hospital Planning,* such as the Jackson County Isolation Hospital in Jackson, Michigan, the Greenville Hospital in Greenville, Maine, and the Royal Victoria Hospital. According to a book review published in 1948, Butler wrote the book for "the use of architects who are called on to plan hospitals, not alone for the man who has never planned one, but also for the architect with experience in the hospital field, for he will realize that something can always be learned from the experience of others."[14] The authors were a good illustration of this counsel. Butler and his coauthor, architect Addison Erdman, "respectfully and affectionately" dedicated the 1946 edition of their popular book to Sigismund Schulz Goldwater, the physician and commissioner of New York City's hospitals from 1934 to 1940 and Stevens.

Edward Palmer York and Philip Sawyer's *Specifications for a Hospital* (1927) was unique among these books in that it was actually the architects' specifications for a hospital they designed in West Chester, Pennsylvania. Intended to serve as a model for other architects, the volume appeared in a series covering the specifications of various building types published by the journal *Pencil Points* (precursor to *Progressive Architecture*). Although their books had markedly different objectives, Stevens and Lee's and York and Sawyer's hospitals looked remarkably similar.[15] The architects may have also met when York and Sawyer designed the stunning Royal Bank building in Montreal in 1928, one of the city's pioneering office buildings.[16]

Networking

Although Stevens actually coauthored only one essay with a physician (the 1911 article with Dr. J. N. E. Brown discussed earlier), he relied on a sophisticated network of physician contacts as consultants. The first two editions of his book were dedicated to Warren Leverne Babcock, the superintendent of the Grace Hospital in Detroit, "whose encouragement and advice decided the writer of this book to devote his entire practice to institutions for the sick." Stevens had designed an addition to the Grace Hospital some time prior to 1913.[17] By the third edition, Stevens had added James Cameron Connell, the dean of medicine at Queen's University in Kingston, Ontario, to Babcock's name. Significantly, Stevens added "in the United States and Canada" to the dedication.

Stevens's opportunity to gain Canadian commissions was no doubt considerably expanded through his association with Brown, and augmented through the partnership he formed with Frederick Clare Lee in 1912 and the opening of their office in Toronto.[18] Lee was born in Chicago in 1874, educated at Yale University and the École des Beaux-Arts (1897–1902), and had moved to Canada in 1907.[19] There he joined the firm of Darling & Pearson, and presumably gained considerable hospital experience with them, since he worked on the Toronto General Hospital (1907–13). Perhaps Brown was responsible for bringing together Stevens and Lee. In 1911–12, Lee practiced independently and was the architect for the Wellesley Hospital in Toronto.[20]

The success of the Stevens and Lee partnership can be measured in the sheer volume of their practice. They designed more than one hundred prominent hospitals in their twenty-one-year partnership.[21] Their monopoly on Canadian hospitals, at least, was uncontested. In 1935, one Canadian intern in five would have trained in a Stevens and Lee–designed building.[22] Just ten years after founding their office, they were at the top of their field in both the United States and Canada. In 1923, Stevens was chosen as the delegate from the American Institute of Architects to the eight hundredth anniversary of the founding of Saint Bartholomew's Hospital in London, England. There he was presented with a medal by the Prince of Wales.[23] Canadian architects admired the firm, too. In 1926, Stevens and Lee won the award for the best hospital from the Ontario Association of Architects.[24]

Staff members were also considered experts in their own rights. Harold Smith, a partner at Stevens and Lee, left the firm and entered into a successful partnership with Canadian architect B. Evan Parry in 1932 in Toronto. British-born Parry had been the director of hospital advisory services to the Canadian government from 1919 to 1932.[25] He published a series of informative articles on hospital architecture in the *Journal of the Royal Architectural Institute of Canada* in the 1930s, intended to serve as reference works to Canadian architects. These articles featured the projects of Stevens and Lee, among others, including large-scale site plans of the hospitals in Ottawa, Kingston, and Montreal. Parry's department also hosted a series of exhibitions of hospital architecture, publicizing the work of his architectural colleagues, and he frequently reported on international conferences for the *Royal Architectural Institute of Canada Journal.* Interestingly, he was also responsible for the "Your Home" column in *Chatelaine,* the popular Canadian women's magazine.[26]

Like his partner, Smith was wholly committed to the new notion of specialized design expertise and took every opportunity to disqualify generalist architects. "It will be readily seen that an architect who has planned a number of such institutions can be of great service to any committee, the average member of which never develops more than one hospital in his life," he told readers of *The Canadian Hospital* in 1925.[27] On at least one occasion, Smith used his experience at Stevens and Lee to lure clients from his former employers. In 1932, he wrote to the superintendent of the Royal Vic proposing Parry and Smith as hospital consultants for the new Montreal Neurological Institute. To ensure that "the building should be most modern in every respect, and generally speaking, the last word in buildings of this type," Smith offered his new firm's services. "Of myself, I need not speak, as I had the pleasure of designing and supervising the work done by my old firm for your institution."[28] He also pointed to the role of Stevens and Lee as consultants. "I would refer to the McGill University Pathological Pavilion which was designed by Messrs. Nobbs and Hyde, the Architects, and for which my old firm Stevens & Lee were consultants for the interior planning and equipment. The desirability of such collaboration is emphasized by the results achieved in this case," explained Smith.[29]

And like Stevens and Lee, the new firm pointed to its investment in travel and the direct observation of numerous institutions as arguments in its favor. Parry's experience with the federal government presumably helped the firm's case as well. Smith noted in his letter to hospital superintendent W. R. Chenoweth that his partner had made "an intensive study of mental institutions throughout this continent for the Dominion Council of Health and has in his possession certain data of great value which is not in the hands of any other architect in Canada."[30]

THE OFFICE

Since Stevens and Lee's papers are not extant, we have no way of knowing how the office actually worked or grew. Stevens and Lee presumably strengthened the firm's breadth of expertise, however, by hiring nonarchitectural specialists, such as Minnie Goodnow. From the tone of her articles, she seems also to have acted as a sort of mediator between the hospital staffs, particularly nurses, and the architects. She was a registered nurse and a former hospital superintendent who subsequently worked in the architects' Boston office as a specialist in hospital equipment. She also authored articles on utility rooms, hospital planning, and hospital details.[31] Goodnow's particular expertise was carefully defined in terms in keeping with those of women architects practicing at this time: interiors, finishes, and detailing. And like many women architects, she defended her own specialization by comparing it to fashion: "A knowledge of plumbing and painting was not harder to acquire than a knowledge of silks or clothes," she stated in 1913.[32] Stevens thanked Goodnow for "work in editing" in the third edition of *The American Hospital of the Twentieth Century*, illuminating yet another responsibility of his female colleague.

Another factor in Stevens's growing professional stature was his significant role as a civilian (nonmilitary) expert with the Engineering Department of the U.S. Army designing overseas hospitals (with Charles Butler) during World War I. In both the original and 1921 editions of his book, Stevens used the opportunity to reproduce the plans of war hospitals by Butler, and those he and Butler had designed together. In the original edition, Stevens noted that the book's publication had even been delayed for a few weeks in order to include the wartime institutions.[33] Stevens, Butler, and L. M. Franklin (of York & Sawyer) later served on a committee to revise army hospitals; Stevens published articles prolifically during this period.

World War I provided Stevens with the first opportunity to design several new related building types, thereby expanding his repertoire of hospital design, such as the Connaught Laboratories at the University of Toronto and the I.O.D.E. (Imperial Order of the Daughters of the Empire, a charitable women's organization) Preventorium (Figure 4.6), also in Toronto. The Connaught Laboratories, unique in Canada at the time, were designed by Stevens and Lee's Toronto office in 1915 and opened in 1917. The labs were intended to produce medical serums, antitoxins, and other products "of a preventive or curative nature" to fight diphtheria, tetanus, and spinal meningitis, and to distribute these free of charge to soldiers (Canadian, French, and British) and civilians.[34]

The Connaught Laboratories were located about ten miles north of Toronto (at Fisherville). The two buildings, constructed of tile and slate, included staff residences, labs, and accommodation for animals.[35] Stevens's aesthetic references in the buildings were clearly rural. A photo of the buildings (Figure 4.7) shows forms inspired by the largely domestic English Arts and Crafts architects, such as C. F. A. Voysey. The Arts and Crafts aesthetic was generally popular in Canada, visible in the work of architects

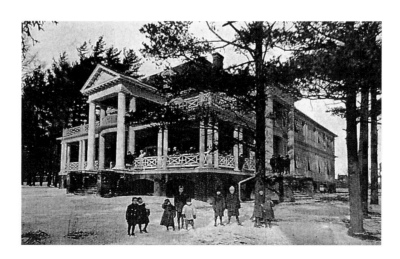

FIGURE 4.6.
I.O.D.E. Preventorium,
Toronto, was for
children suspected of
having tuberculosis.

such as Eden Smith in Toronto and Percy Nobbs in Montreal.[36] The horses, which were bled to produce the antitoxins, were "housed" in the larger building, a U-shaped structure with a steeply gabled roof and off-center tower.[37] Perhaps the architectural references to large country houses made sense to Stevens, too, because the fifty-acre farm on which the labs were located was the gift of Colonel Albert E. Gooderham.[38] For the interior of the avant-garde labs, however, Stevens looked to the factory for inspiration, rather than to the home.

The Connaught Laboratories received wide coverage in the press for their heroic work in medicine. The research done at the lab was compared to that of the Lister Institute, the Pasteur Institute, and the Rockefeller Institute.[39] And the Ontario government's decision to distribute its products at reduced prices or even free put the province "in the van in public health work."[40] Presumably its architects, too, would have shared in this attention. Similarly, Stevens and Lee's design for the I.O.D.E. Preventorium was on the cutting edge of preventive medicine. The plan (Figure 4.8) featured a two-story sleeping veranda and adjacent exterior verandas, for children to play. The overall function of the building was to carefully observe children suspected of having tuberculosis.

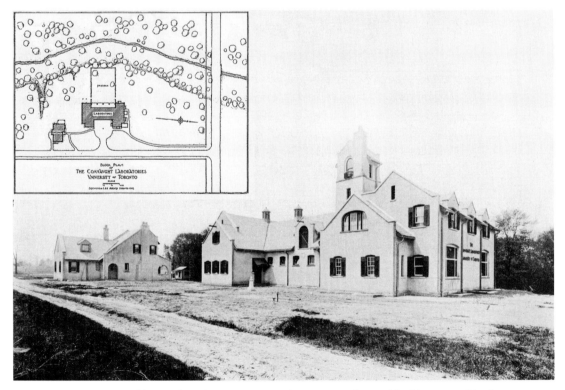

FIGURE 4.7. World War I brought opportunities for innovative hospital building types like the Connaught Laboratories, which produced medical products for soldiers.

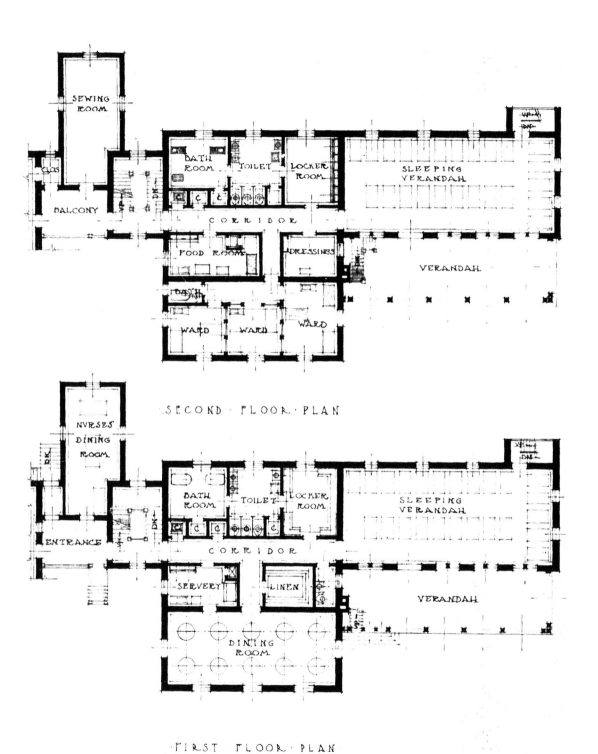

SEWING
ROOM

CLOS

BALCONY

BATH
ROOM

TOILET

LOCKER
ROOM

SLEEPING
VERANDAH

CORRIDOR

FOOD ROOM

DRESSING

VERANDAH

BATH

WARD

WARD

WARD

SECOND · FLOOR · PLAN

NURSES'
DINING
ROOM

DN

ENTRANCE

DN

BATH
ROOM

TOILET

LOCKER
ROOM

SLEEPING
VERANDAH

CORRIDOR

SERVERY

LINEN

VERANDAH

DINING
ROOM

FIRST · FLOOR · PLAN

FIGURE 4.8. I.O.D.E. Preventorium, plan.

There is one other important measure of the firm's influence just after the war and the publication of *The American Hospital of the Twentieth Century*. Stevens and Lee's commission in 1919 for Montreal's Hôpital Notre-Dame (whose architecture is explored in chapter 5) is a good illustration of their distinguished professional stature at this time. Bucking the tradition of French Catholic architects for French Catholic hospitals, the committee apparently hired Stevens because it wanted an up-to-date, modernized hospital.

Although the hiring of Stevens for this francophone hospital was significant, it is only one aspect of a larger shift that saw Canadian hospital administrators in general move from a reliance on European models in the nineteenth century, to American ones after about 1900, another pattern still in evidence today. Perhaps this crucial shift occurred because the practice of twentieth-century Canadian medicine was closer to the American model, especially as ties in medical education to places like Edinburgh grew weaker with subsequent generations. But it also may be due, at least in part, to the dominance of Stevens and Lee as hospital architects.

Learning from Observing

Stevens's expertise was based on three areas of experience and knowledge. Firstly, his familiarity with the equipment and techniques of medicine and surgery; secondly, his understanding of the equipment and techniques of the institution's kitchen, laundry, and powerhouse; and thirdly, his awareness of cost-efficient, practical construction. The first two areas of knowledge Stevens derived from decades of close observation of hospital practice, rather than from book learning. In 1945, two years after his retirement, Stevens articulated the qualifications of a specialized hospital architect. He urged young architects studying to become hospital specialists to "visualize everything that goes on in the institution." He suggested that the best experience would come from "a long series of visits, oft repeated, to institutions known to be satisfactory, whose reputations can be verified," in which architects could observe doctors, nurses, and nonprofessionals, undertake time studies, watch surgeries, read books, interview department heads, and even observe autopsies.[41]

This emphasis on suggested reforms through personal observation echoes the celebrated work of Florence Nightingale, who professionalized nursing following her first-hand experience of military hospitals during the Crimean War in the 1850s. Equally famous is the work of Frederick Winslow Taylor, a contemporary of Stevens's, who observed individual laborers at work in the field, set up a series of experiments, and observed relations between management and labor toward his theory of scientific management.[42]

Designer Doctors

Just as Stevens developed considerable expertise in matters medical, some physicians became experts in architectural design. Hospital expert Burdett, whose medical education was actually incomplete, was "constantly consulted about new hospitals . . . from the time of Johns Hopkins Hospital and before that, down to now."[43] For Burdett, this legacy was carried on in North America by Goldwater, who acted as "advisory construction expert" for 156 hospitals.[44] Physicians like Goldwater were central to the burgeoning constellation of hospital experts that developed in the interwar period, and threatened the need for specialist architects. Could not any architect who could organize and incorporate the work of consultants design a hospital?

The hospital architect actually had to please a new breed of hospital managers, administrators, regulators, and consultants in the early twentieth century. These individuals were not necessarily interested in the details of the medical practices; they saw the hospital in all of its functional and technological complexity and were thus quite distinct from the laypeople who now patronized the institution. Nonspecialized administrators typically had their own, generally nontechnical, expectations of what a hospital should be.[45]

In the interwar period, physicians like Goldwater with expertise in planning and construction were typically hired to assist, and in some cases, even to police the architect. Goldwater worked on at least five major hospitals in Canada: the Montreal General Hospital, the Jewish General Hospital in Montreal, the Vancouver General Hospital, the Toronto Western Hospital, and the Hamilton General Hospital. He also met with Ernest Cormier over the design of the Université de Montréal, presumably in his capacity as an outspoken advocate of the "vertical" hospital.[46]

Physician William Henry Walsh, consultant to the Hamilton General, the General Public Hospital in St. John, New Brunswick, and St. Mary's Hospital in Montreal, teamed up with architect-engineer Edgar Martin. In 1932, they suggested that the "combined experience of the authors" validated their suggestions regarding hospital planning and construction. Perhaps most significant in their article, which they claimed to be "a radical departure from the orthodox and time-honored approach to the subject," was Walsh and Martin's articulation of the hospital architect's "cognitive exclusiveness" and their reiteration, echoing Stevens, that it was the complexity of the hospital plan that required specialized architects:

> A hospital is not like any other building. It is an intricate and involved building operation in which, contrary to the usual practice, the architect is unable to commence his labors by the establishment of an exterior design. On the contrary, his ingenuity is taxed to the limit in an endeavor to conform facades and elevations of symmetry and beauty, without waste or architectural superfluities, to a predetermined interior layout over which he has little control. The engineering features of a hospital, both structural and mechanical, are so involved and the design so complicated that the architect who is successful in obtaining low building costs, and incidentally low operating costs, must possess that degree of skill that will enable him to approach the problem from the functional standpoint, delaying the study of elevations and architectural exterior until floor plans are well worked out.[47]

Like Stevens's position in architecture, Goldwater's position in the new field of "hospital consultant" was virtually uncontested. The qualifications of such a consultant were also clearly described in Walsh and Martin's 1932 article:

> The place of the medical consultant in a hospital building program has been definitely fixed for all time by the distinguished pioneer activities of Dr. Goldwater, whose accomplishments have been so preeminent that few have been able to follow the standards he has set. The qualifications of a hospital consultant are exacting and his success depends upon his ability to coordinate and apply all available information bearing upon a particular project, to thoroughly understand all of the technical details of professional service, and to transmit and interpret these to the architect in an intelligent manner. That the value of a competent consultant, conversant alike with the intricate problems of the professional services and with the fundamentals of building construction, is attested by the fact that today few informed sponsors of new hosptials can be induced to undertake such projects without this expert guidance. . . . As for the attitude of the architects, it may be said without exaggeration that the more experience they accumulate in this type of work, the more enthusiastically do they favor the collaboration of a competent medical aid[e]. There can be no conflict between the consultant and the architect when each knows his business and recognizes his limitations.[48]

Goldwater's and Stevens's professional paths must have intersected frequently. Certainly their names appear on the same programs for major conferences and meetings. Perhaps they met over their mutual interests in the development of the Royal Victoria Hospital. While Stevens's participation in the design of the Montreal buildings was continuous and ongoing, however, Goldwater served the hospital only once: during the design of the Montreal Neurological Institute, located just east of the Royal Victoria Hospital.

Controversies

Two issues distinguished Stevens from most of his hospital architect colleagues. Physicians were quick to criticize him for his preference for daylit surgical suites and Europe-derived penchant for hydrotherapy facilities. As already mentioned, Stevens became an avid supporter of hydrotherapy following his careful study of European hospitals with Brown in 1911.[49] In their co-designed one-hundred-bed hospital published just following their European tour, the architect-physician duo included hydrotherapy and "electric treatment" facilities directly adjacent to the medical wards, reminding readers that such therapies "bear somewhat the same relation to the medical service as the operating suite does to the surgical."[50] Three years later, Stevens presented his rather controversial support for hydro- and other paramedical therapies in a paper at the annual conference of the American Hospital Association, in St. Paul, Minnesota. In "The Need of Better

Hospital Equipment for the Medical Man," Stevens illustrated how American hospitals provided state-of-the-art facilities for the surgeon, while ignoring the needs of medical experts. German hospitals, Stevens argued, provided a better balance, giving ample space to electro-, hydro-, dry heat, light, and mechanotherapies.[51] More than a decade later, in 1926, Stevens stated that "the careful student of hospital architecture will not dare to plan his buildings without providing facilities for these medical treatments."[52] By then, however, the tremendous casualties during World War I had increased the public's and physicians' confidence in such treatments.[53]

By this time, too, Stevens could hold up his own designs for the Ross Pavilion at the Royal Victoria Hospital and the Ottawa Civic Hospital, both of which included hydrotherapy facilities (Figure 4.9), as model buildings in this regard. Stevens included a detailed plan of the Ross medical department in the second, but not the first edition of his book; in the third edition, he included a photo of the hydrotherapeutic room at the Ottawa Civic Hospital and wrote that the facility there was "not elaborate, but is fairly complete," suggesting that it may have met an acceptable minimum standard.[54]

His opinions concerning the natural illumination of surgical suites were similarly controversial, and were particularly unpopular with surgeons. They sometimes did not

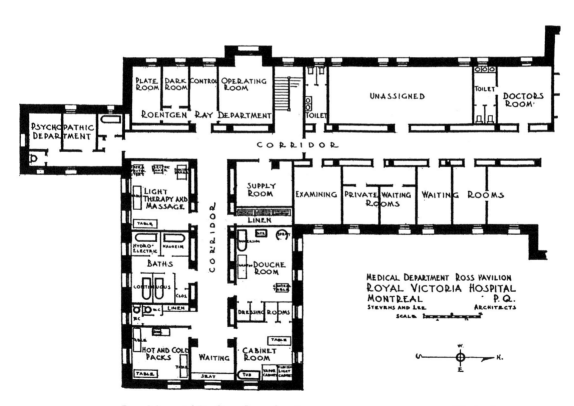

FIGURE 4.9. Ross Memorial Pavilion, floor plan. Stevens was a strong proponent of hydrotherapy and always advocated space for baths in his hospitals.

bother arguing with Stevens, but instead covered up the large windows he specified for operating rooms, in some cases soon after the building opened. A signature of Stevens's hospitals were, in fact, large floor-to-ceiling windows that met a skylight or angled window at the ceiling, providing surgeons with both side and top lighting; several examples of this detail were included in his book, such as the operating rooms at Bridgeport Hospital, Barre City Hospital, and Young & Hall's Hospital of St. John and Elizabeth, in London, England.[55]

Doctors' dislike of large windows started long before Stevens's era. A photograph of the Pemberton Memorial Operating Theatre from 1897 shows the windows partially whitewashed, perhaps offering surgeons a combination of artificial and natural light (Figure 4.10). Most surgeons, however, in the interwar period preferred artificial lighting in the operating room. They pointed to the variability of daylight in terms of both quality and color; complained that they could not control the direction of natural light; and emphasized the power savings to be gleaned from designing a system of illumination that could be tailored to the precise needs of each surgical procedure.[56] Artificial lighting was considered more "scientific" than natural illumination.[57]

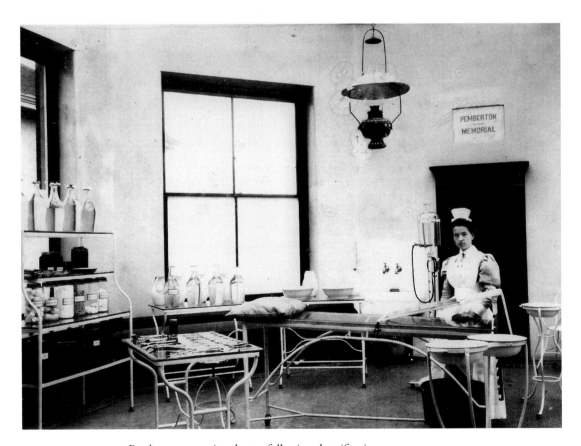

FIGURE 4.10. Pemberton operating theater following electrification.

The Ottawa Civic Hospital serves as a particularly good example of Stevens's commitment to both hydrotherapy and naturally lit operating rooms, even in the face of medical opposition.[58] It also illustrates how existing hospitals, both designed in isolation and as additions, served as models for new design and justified the hiring of experts. Stevens and Lee were engaged by the hospital during their busy postwar, postbook years, in October 1919. Driving the boom in hospital construction during these years was the worldwide influenza epidemic, which swept Canada in 1918, during which thousands of Canadians had direct experience of severe illness and became keenly aware of the need for hospital facilities.

The Ottawa Civic Hospital (OCH) was under construction from 1920 to 1924, opening on November 27, 1924. Originally intended to accommodate six hundred patients, Stevens's design for the new hospital was a monumental, six-story, H-shaped redbrick building. Its monumentality was due mostly to its scale and to its rather imposing white stone entrance, which featured four gigantic Corinthian columns (three stories high). Behind the main building, and connected by means of tunnels, were a smaller service building, female help building, powerhouse, and garage. Directly west of the administration building and separated by a tunnel, was Stevens and Lee's 230-room residence for nurses. All the buildings were set in a parklike, elevated, twenty-four-acre site, framed by curving paths and picturesque plantings. An enclosed porte cochere at the rear of the main building anticipated delivery of patients by ambulance and car.[59] This feature was particularly important, given that the hospital was located on the outskirts of the city, reflecting the general post–World War I trend toward "a programme of exteriorization."[60]

In all likelihood, Stevens's earlier job at the Ross Memorial Pavilion at the Royal Victoria Hospital in Montreal in 1916 led to his being hired in Ottawa. Indeed, the Ross seems to have served as something of a showpiece for Stevens, perhaps because of its visibility as one of the earliest paying patients' pavilions. He published a model of the building and two floor plans in the second of two significant articles in the influential journal, *Architectural Record*, while the Ross was under construction in 1916.

There is evidence, too, that members of the OCH board visited other hospitals by Stevens and Lee around this time, including the Children's Hospital in Halifax, the Hospital for Sick Children in Toronto, and the Isolation Hospital in Toronto. Hospital superintendents were closely connected through an organized network, which was probably an important conduit for information on good architects and good building materials.[61] At least one letter was sent to administrators responsible for the Montreal private-patients' hospital to inquire about Stevens's performance.[62]

By far the most important model for the Ottawa Civic Hospital, however, was the Cincinnati General Hospital, described by J. H. W. Bower in a report read before the hospital board, following his visit to the building during the American Hospital Association meeting there in 1916.[63] Stevens, too, praised the Cincinnati institution (especially its choice of site) in *The American Hospital of the Twentieth Century*, as well as the thorough study of precedents made by medical adviser Christian R. Holmes.[64]

Stevens made sure to include the Cincinnati building, along with his own, in the slide presentation he made to the OCH trustees in March 1920. In a letter to the hospital superintendent written days before the presentation, he reiterated his authority as a hospital designer and suggested how his lantern slides of "numerous large hospitals throughout the world" shown to "a large body of people" may serve as a critical context for his own work: "I can point out to the people just how our plan differs from almost any hospital in the country, and I think it will appear to advantage in contrast with the others."[65]

Conclusion

The ways in which Stevens established expertise were different from those of the experts who came just before him, and directly linked to the practice of medicine. As we have seen in chapter 1, architects practicing before about 1900, such as Henry Saxon Snell and the other major designers of the pavilion-plan hospital at its height, established their hospital expertise through their vast experience in designing and constructing other institutions for social reform (prisons, schools, workhouses, almshouses, asylums, and orphanages), which, like hospitals, were largely benevolent institutions with complex programmatic requirements. There is no indication whatsoever in the primary sources that these architects saw the design of the "nonplan" aspects of the hospital as a separate, less difficult responsibility; and they often resented the hiring of local, nonspecialized architects to supervise their work.

This is not so with architects after about 1900. This next generation, that is, architects like Stevens and his colleagues, bolstered their architectural authority not through their experience building related institutions, but rather through their direct observation of medical practice.[66] It was their special knowledge of the routines, needs, and procedures of specific departments that enabled them to master the complex programmatic requirements of the modern hospital.

A significant result of this direct observation of international medical practice resulted in professional tensions. These extended beyond lighting surgical rooms and providing hydrotherapy departments. Location, site conditions, parking, entrance design (separate or not), balancing domestic comfort with institutional hygiene, and dozens of other issues were debated in the built environment. Hospital architecture, then as now, was fiercely contested. Like all buildings, they are dynamic products of widely varying ideals.

Modernisms

THIS FINAL CHAPTER EXPLORES THE ARCHITECTURE OF EDWARD F. Stevens and his partner, Frederick Clare Lee, during the 1920s, a critical period of expansion in the history of the North American hospital. Stevens and Lee's work is representative here of a whole wave of modern institutions that incorporated and promoted social and medical change. Driven by the changes and tensions outlined in chapters 2, 3, and 4, the key features of the modern institutions included historicist imagery, steel and reinforced concrete framing, fireproofing, soundproofing, functional zoning, overt references to domestic and hotel architecture, delivery by automobile, internal communication technologies, adherence to standards, planning for expansion, factory-inspired kitchens and laundries, suites of rooms for surgery, and a new emphasis on individual patient rooms. Designed by experts with personal knowledge of outstanding doctors and their preferred work settings, Stevens and Lee's buildings set a new North American standard.

HISTORICIST IMAGERY, MODERN MEDICINE

Modern hospitals during the 1920s combined technological fetishism with intense social conservatism. Architects evoked historical styles and used traditional materials for the conservative outside of their buildings, while finding multiple and often ingenious ways to incorporate and display technologically advanced medical, service, and managerial equipment inside. Stevens and Lee's Hôpital Notre-Dame's exterior, for example, was "hard burned rough textured buff brick."[1] The Montreal hospital's main entrance featured double-height Corinthian columns (Figure 5.1) of Stanstead granite and a segmented arch. The building had a pronounced base and cornice, quoins of Montreal limestone, and its windows had keystones. These classical details—"all trim and special architectural features"—ensured that Hôpital Notre-Dame, an urban institution, was decorously comforting and dignified.

Just as he camouflaged mechanical equipment in the medieval-styled tower of the Ross Memorial Pavilion at the Royal Vic, Stevens cloaked particularly high-tech departments of Hôpital Notre-Dame in traditional exterior features. At the back of the romantic arcade on the ground floor of the new hospital was the department for otolaryngology (ear, nose, and throat). Surgery was similarly camouflaged, but prominently featured in

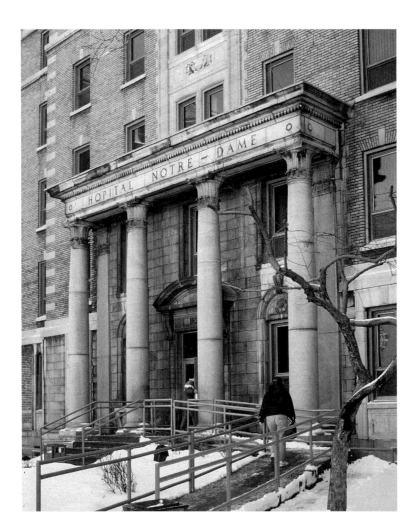

FIGURE 5.1.
Stevens and Lee's
entrance to Hôpital
Notre-Dame featured
classical columns.

this same elevation (Figure 5.2). Two large windows located just over the cornice line call attention to the surgical wing.[2]

Behind such historicist guises, North American hospitals constructed in the 1920s were thoroughly modern. Both Hôpital Notre-Dame and Stevens's Ottawa Civic Hospital (Figure 5.3) were reinforced concrete frames with combination brick and tile curtain walls. In addition, the arrangement of girders and columns meant that the reinforced concrete structure of the Stevens and Lee hospitals could also carry the pipes and ducts for the gravity exhaust ventilation system. Stevens's structural system supported the mechanical design, which was integrated with functional zoning; this meant that a specific department could be ventilated independently by pushing a button from within the department.[3]

In the 1920s, hospitals were designed as thoroughly fireproof and older buildings modernized for fire protection. This desire for safety inspired architects to specify incombustible materials (concrete floors) separated by hollow terra cotta tiles, brick and stone cladding, partitions of terra cotta tile, gypsum tile or plaster on metal lath.[4] In his book, Stevens admitted that the doors, windows, furnishings, and linen might be combustible, for as "to have them otherwise would make them so ugly and impractical as to more than offset the slight menace of fire."[5]

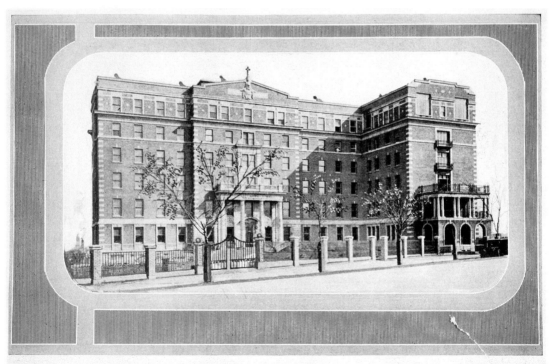

LA FACADE DU NOUVEL HOPITAL NOTRE-DAME, RUE SHERBROOKE

FIGURE 5.2. High-tech departments like surgery were subtly visible in the facade of Hôpital Notre-Dame.

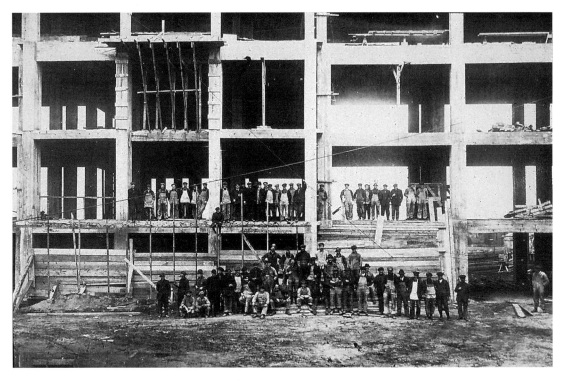

FIGURE 5.3. Ottawa Civic Hospital under construction, 1922–23.

Urban Problems and the Hospital

The effects of modernity in other domains were explicitly addressed in Stevens's architecture. Stevens, for example, took special care to buffer the loud noises produced outside the hospital, especially those of automobiles (he noted the honking and starting of cars), airplanes, trains, and streetcars. The new noisy machinery of urban transportation ironically also helped hospitals perform better. Automobiles and paved roads meant that urgent patients would arrive sooner; doctors could reach the hospital quickly from their clinics, offices, and homes; and medicine, food, and other supplies could be delivered to the hospital more efficiently. Stevens's projects such as the Ottawa Civic Hospital that were not additions or renovations to older sites were frequently located at some distance from the city center in order to simultaneously take advantage of motor tranportation and escape the noise and pollution of the urban core.

Noise control was a major factor in the planning of hospitals. For Stevens, soundproofing was a way to tolerate rather than resist urban crowding, which was necessary to the economic health of hospitals. Stevens recommended locating serving kitchens in cross-corridors, rather than corridors leading to the patients' rooms, in order to minimize noise transmission.[6] Such noise, as well as bad smells, was particularly unacceptable to middle-class patients, willing to pay for private (and thus quieter) rooms. This acoustic and olfactory control fits with the range of other luxuries we encountered in such buildings in chapter 2.

Ironically, it was modern construction and planning that created these noise problems in the hospital. Noisy corridors were a new problem created by the double-loaded plan arrangement combined with fireproof construction. The multitude of smaller rooms located on both sides of a narrow corridor (as opposed to the open wards of the pavilion-plan hospital with minimal circulation spaces) meant that hospital specifications included hundreds of doors, opening and closing at all times of day and night. Telephones and call systems rang constantly, disturbing patients and staff.[7] Stair towers and elevators were carefully located away from patient rooms, often on side corridors.

Servicing more rooms, too, meant that hallways would become congested with staff and equipment. Strict visiting hours were enforced in order to make hospitals quieter, and management likewise urged nurses and interns to minimize their socializing: "Even after nurses pass the probationary period, if they persist in disturbing the wards by engaging in foolish talking and laughing with house surgeons or visitors they should be severely reprimanded."[8]

To muffle sounds produced within the hospital—plumbing, signal bells, doors and windows slamming, and patients talking—Stevens recommended doors "with special gaskets," "pipes and vent ducts wrapped with heavy felt," acoustic plaster in corridors and service rooms, and sound-absorbing Celotex ceilings in especially noisy spaces: serveries, utility rooms, and the delivery suite.[9] Stevens and Lee's St. Joseph's Hospital in Toronto (Figure 5.4) featured "sound stopping" gypsum partition tiles. Stevens also claimed to have patented the soundproofing treatment he devised for the Royal Victoria Montreal Maternity Hospital in 1925 (Figure 5.5), a focus of chapter 2.[10] It was called the "Stevens System" and featured what he called "Stevens isolators" and "Stevens low felted chairs" in walls and ceilings. Stevens suggested in *Modern Hospital* in 1925 that the time might soon come for the hospital to put a sign up on its chimney "for the aeronaut to read as he passes by—'Hospital Zone! Shut off the motor while passing!'"[11]

The debate on the health benefits of the so-called block plan, this arrangement of smaller rooms along double-loaded corridors, over the older pavilion-plan type raged during the two decades of Stevens and Lee's practice, focusing on the question of how to balance the efficiency and economy of the ward with the comfort and protection of the private room.[12] Some physicians claimed that the total spatial separation of patients would curb the spread of contagious diseases, while other social commentators, even Henry Ford, argued that private rooms were more democratic.[13] To some extent, the same sociomedical debates continue today.

Stevens walked the line between the two sides of the debate, professing a middle-ground solution for the middle-class patient (the poor continued to occupy wards, while the rich paid for private space) and pointing to the subdivided wards of two Danish hospitals as models. He typically provided wards for sixteen to eighteen patients, in groups

QUIET HOSPITALS
Are a Question of Technical Study Leading to
SOUND ABSORPTION
SOUND STOPPING

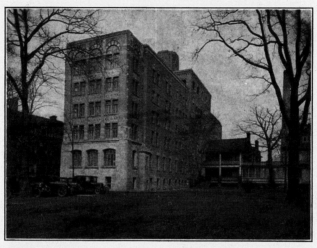

St. Joseph's Hospital,
Toronto, Ont.

Architects—Stevens and Lee.
Contractors—Pigott Construction Co.

In this building 60,000 square feet of Gypsum Partition Tile were installed to provide permanently fire-proof partitions between rooms. This application of Gypsum has prevented sound passing from room to room in the building.

Taking advantage of the consulting services of Prof. G. R. Anderson, of the University of Toronto, DEKOOSTO Acoustic Plaster was used to absorb sound within the building. By this medium it was possible to instal exactly the proper amount of acoustic treatment in every room in the building where it was needed, and to know in advance the results which would be obtained.

A complete consulting service on problems of fire, sound and heat insulation is available to the building public in Canada to-day without charge. A call to any office or representative will place this at the disposal of any building owner, architect or contractor.

GYPSUM, LIME & ALABASTINE,
CANADA, LIMITED
HEAD OFFICE   -   PARIS, ONTARIO
BRANCHES: MONTREAL, TORONTO, WALKERVILLE, WINNIPEG, VANCOUVER

FIGURE 5.4. Advertisement for gypsum partition tiles featuring a hospital designed by Stevens and Lee.

of three or four "alcove" wards, recommending that each patient be allotted from eighty-three to one hundred square feet of floor area and a floor-to-ceiling height of twelve feet.[14] This smallish ward, Stevens believed, would satisfy "the great intermediate class of patients who, with the 'ward pocketbook,' are acquiring the 'private room appetite.'"[15] Hospitals boasted that the thin, metal partitions that separated patients in such wards served to even out differences in social class, as well as separating potentially dangerous patients. The Montreal Jewish General Hospital, for example, featured four-bed public wards and boasted that the food and furniture were identical for public and private patients.[16]

While thin metal walls blurred social distinctions among patients, Stevens's choice of flooring materials expressed the spatial separation of functions. The interwar hospital was planned in functional zones, very much like the modern city, and the hospital's flooring materials were carefully matched to the various functions of spaces, reflecting then current notions in acoustics and cleaning, but also denoting the social hierarchy of certain spaces. Wards and patients' rooms typically had sound-absorbing floor coverings, such as linoleum (Figure 5.6), cork, or rubber.[17] The last was also recommended for the floors and ceilings of X-ray departments.[18] The floors of balconies, waiting rooms, and kitchens were covered in quarry tile; vitreous tile was found on the floors of operating rooms.

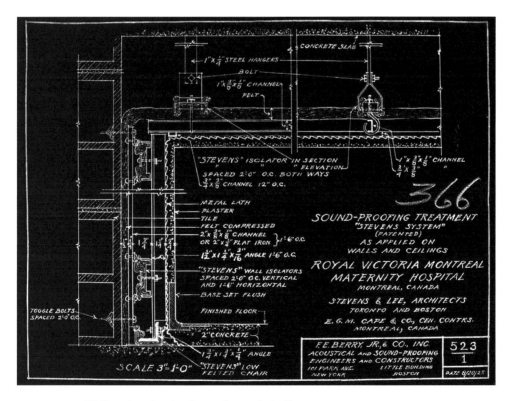

FIGURE 5.5. Wall section showing Stevens's soundproofing system, 1925.

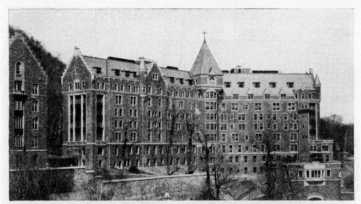

New Maternity Wing of the Royal Victoria Hospital, Montreal, in the halls and wards of which Dominion Jaspé Linoleum was used extensively.

Architects—Stevens & Lee, Toronto.   Contractor—E. G. M. Cape & Co., Montreal.

Quiet, Permanent Floors

IT IS of the utmost importance that the floors of a hospital be quiet, odorless and durable. These same qualities are also of prime importance in selecting the floors for any building. Dominion Battleship Linoleum is a permanent floor. It is so tough that the hardest usage, year after year, has no effect on it. There is no replacement cost with Dominion Battleship Linoleum. An occasional waxing meets the needs of those who prefer a highly polished floor.

DOMINION
Battleship Linoleum

The smooth surface of Dominion Battleship Linoleum will not absorb moisture or hold dirt; it is germicidal; odorless even in hottest weather; easily cleaned. By silent service it has answered the floor problem in banks, offices, hospitals, department stores, libraries and public institutions in every Province of the Dominion.

Dominion Battleship Linoleum, AAA quality, is made in eight standard shades—brown, green, terra cotta, grey, buff, blue, black and white (used extensively for tile floors). AA and A qualities, in four standard shades only: Dominion Jaspé, 1st and 3rd grades, in two colours only—blue and grey. Special colours for large contracts.

Dominion Battleship Linoleum is made in Canada to suit Canada's climatic conditions and is installed by all large departmental and house furnishing stores. Write us for free samples and literature.

Dominion Oilcloth & Linoleum Co., Limited
MONTREAL
Makers of Floor Coverings for over Fifty Years.

FIGURE 5.6. Advertisement for Dominion battleship linoleum.

Terrazzo was used throughout the hospital, due to its cheapness and durability, while marble was often reserved for use in the hospital lobby.[19] Indeed, the lobbies in the Ottawa Civic Hospital, Hôpital Notre-Dame, and the pavilions at the Royal Victoria Hospital resembled hotel lobbies, because of their ostentatious materials and historicist decoration. As noted in chapter 2, the lobby at the Ross Pavilion (Figure 5.7), illustrated in *The American Hospital of the Twentieth Century,* was intended as a memorial vestibule to the building's benefactors. John Kenneth Leveson Ross erected it in memory of his parents, James Ross and Annie Kerr Ross. A bronze bust was positioned on axis with the entry, perched on a grand oak-and-marble pedestal, which also functioned to conceal the radiators. Perhaps this rather solemn memorial function of the room persuaded Stevens and Lee to use Caen stone on the walls and groined ceiling of the Ross Pavilion lobby, "depart[ing] from the hospital type of finish."[20] The twenty-six-foot by thirty-two-foot entrance to the Ross Pavilion also had five bronze chandeliers, fine oak paneling, and Belgian-black and Italian-white tile flooring, illustrating Stevens's counsel that the entrance furniture should be both "dignified and decorative."[21]

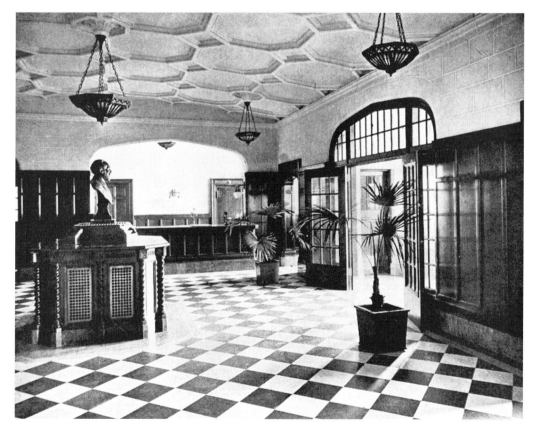

FIGURE 5.7. The lobby of the Ross Memorial Pavilion featured luxurious materials and hotel-like details in order to entice paying patients.

At the same time, many historicist-decorated hospital lobbies, including the Ross Pavilion, anticipated the delivery of patients by automobile (Figure 5.8). In 1916, the Ross Pavilion entry sequence comprised heavy wrought iron gates at the street (see Figure 2.3), a curvilinear driveway rising about one thousand feet, "sufficiently broad to allow the turning of automobiles and carriages," and a porte cochere. The hospital thus not only accommodated new modes of transportation, but by doing so also reinforced the new modes as desirable and permanent. Automobile parking was thus an important feature of the modern hospital. Photographs of the Ottawa Civic Hospital taken about 1924 (Figure 5.9) show Model T Fords parked along the driveway and in designated parking lots (Stevens wanted them located "at some distance" from the patients' rooms). The Ottawa Civic Hospital added a luxurious fourteen-car parking garage (Figure 5.10) for doctors in 1930, which heated the vehicles to a toasty ninety degrees Fahrenheit using excess boiler heat.[22] As early as 1911, the Royal Victoria Hospital had added parking lots for doctors and private patients and a special entrance and garage for its ambulances. This was only a year after Ford opened his advanced car manufacturing plant at Highland Park, Michigan.

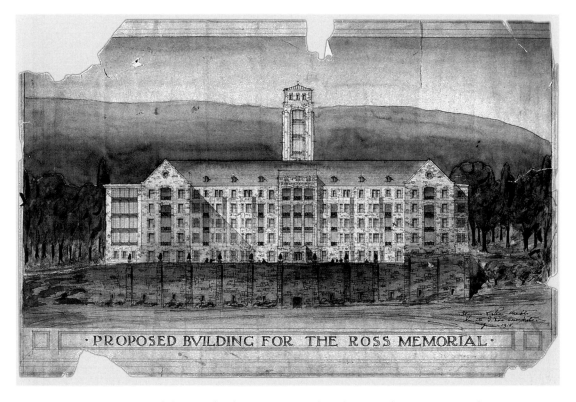

FIGURE 5.8. Proposed elevation for the Ross Memorial Pavilion, Royal Victoria Hospital, 1914.

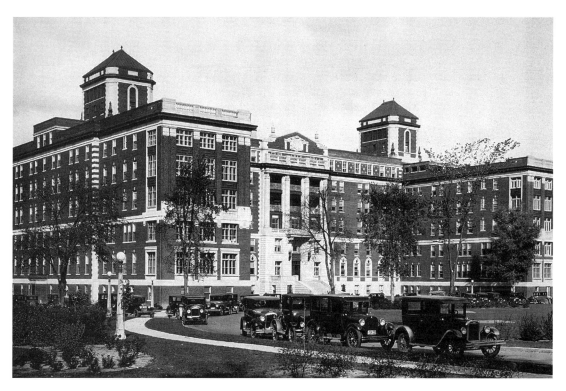

FIGURE 5.9. Ottawa Civic Hospital with cars, 1925.

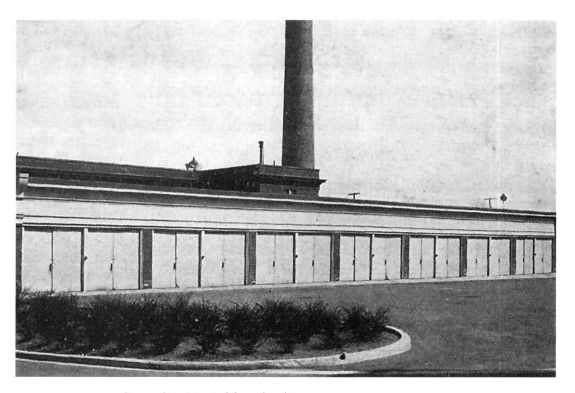

FIGURE 5.10. Ottawa Civic Hospital, heated parking garage.

STANDARDIZATION VERSUS FLEXIBILITY

Stevens took every opportunity to build technology (instrument cabinets, refrigerators, blanket warmers, and drying closets) directly into the hospital walls. The private patients' rooms in the maternity hospital at the Royal Victoria (see Figure 2.15) were wired for telephone and each floor had receptacles for electrocardiograph. Patients' rooms had special night-lights, allowing nurses to illuminate the rooms at night without using ceiling lights, in addition to a call system similar to those found in many hospitals today. This consisted of a system of lights over the doors of rooms indicating the location of doctors and nurses.

These technologies were largely standardized during Stevens's lifetime, a process accelerated by the American experience during World War I.[23] In 1918, the American College of Surgeons developed standards and encouraged hospitals across North America to apply for approval. The ACS published annual lists of hospitals that met its minimum standards, with more and more hospitals satisfying its criteria each year. In 1918, 89 of 697 eligible hospitals with one hundred or more beds met ACS approval; by 1921, this number had increased to 576.[24]

The arguments for the standardization of hospitals were well worn: public safety, cost efficiency, and hospital evaluation. Architects, however, as professionals responsible for custom-designed health-care facilities, occupied an ambivalent position vis-à-vis the standardization of hospital design. Would not the eventual adoption of a standard hospital plan make specialists like Stevens and Lee obsolete? In the 1920s and 1930s, it was not unusual for specialized journals to publish "checklists" of hospital equipment, in order to avoid errors of omission.[25] The lists organized in 1934 for *The Hospital Yearbook* by Sigismund Schulz Goldwater, physician and commissioner of New York City's hospitals from 1934 to 1940, considered the planning of wards, private rooms, and various departments of the hospital.[26] Stevens's book was in some ways the same sort of thing: a checklist of points to consider and standards to uphold in the design of a hospital. Stevens himself advocated the standardization of hospital equipment, pointing to the wartime experience with plumbing as a case in point, but he was completely opposed to the standardization of hospital plans, noting the necessity of judgment in dealing with the complexities of site and circumstances. His book and articles made the same argument by underlining his professional authority (the book showcased his own buildings), offering only the most general guidelines and implying that each commission demanded a unique solution.[27]

Stevens might also have noted how designing for built-in technology and standardization was an impulse contradictory to allowing for both expansion and change. Much of the firm's work involved adding to older buildings, or designing hospitals to be constructed in stages, such as Hôpital Notre-Dame. Only three of the firm's twenty or so Canadian commissions, in fact, were for completely new buildings. Planning for expansion was thus a fundamental aspect of hospital modernization and specialization. It was particularly important in the choice of a site, which had to provide ample space for the hospital's growth, as well as anticipate the way the surrounding city might develop. "In selecting a site it was necessary to have enough land available for future expansion and, at the same time, a location easily accessible to the medical men and patients, as well as one that would be in the path of the city's normal growth," Stevens recounted about the Ottawa Civic Hospital.[28]

He was equally concerned about designing flexible space in his hospitals. In *The American Hospital of the Twentieth Century,* he quoted from Goldwater's report of the Committee on Hospital Planning of 1924, to the American Hospital Association, whose fourth principle was "flexibility." By this Stevens meant far more than facilitating simple, unanticipated alterations, but rather the potential of a building to adapt to a total change in function. He imagined, for example, "a plan so flexible that the medical department of yesterday may be the surgical department of to-morrow."[29]

Although the plans of interwar hospitals consisted of mostly smaller rooms off long, double-loaded corridors, aspects of the earlier pavilion-plan buildings survived in the newer buildings, a fact rarely noted by hospital historians. However, new hospitals of the 1920s included features of both types. Which features of the pavilion-plan hospital were carried into the reformed buildings and why? Like other general hospitals of the 1920s, Stevens's designs nearly always had some sort of ward accommodation for poorer patients, often called "public wards." These were typically smaller than their nineteenth-century precedents; at Hôpital Notre-Dame, for example, the second floor featured square public wards that were forty-three feet wide and contained twenty beds. These spaces were further subdivided into smaller sections containing five beds, separated from the others by partitions that did not quite reach the ceiling.[30]

New Ways of Working

The sophisticated physical structure and features of the modern hospital paralleled an up-to-date social structure: the hospital restructured ways of working. Within his (apparent) Renaissance palazzo or Scottish castle hospitals, Stevens's planning facilitated the working methods of highly specialized physicians, nurses, teams of orderlies and other aides, administrators, janitorial and laundry staffs, all trained to work as efficiently and productively as possible, as we have seen. In addition to the overall arrangement of the building that grouped patients by the general treatment they required, the premium placed on time and efficiency led to the inclusion of nonmedical technology such as time clocks, call systems, and adding machines, then becoming familiar in other modern corporations and institutions.[31]

The quest for efficiency, driven not by medical science but rather by social change, also fashioned a need to improve the performance of existing nonmedical technologies like elevators. A 1927 advertisement for Otis-Fensom elevators (Figure 5.11) featuring the Royal Victoria Hospital boasted that following three years of microleveling elevator

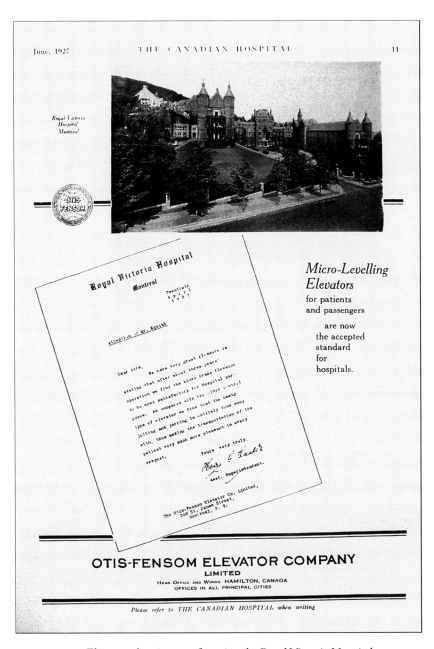

FIGURE 5.11. Elevator advertisement featuring the Royal Victoria Hospital.

operation, "nasty jolting and jarring" had been done away with, making the movement of patients and passenger considerably smoother. Stevens made the same point in *The American Hospital of the Twentieth Century:* "An automatic levelling device is a most important adjunct to a hospital elevator."[32] Elevators only became important when they ran smoothly, which coincided with the time that hospitals became multistory blocks rather than pavilions and patients had to be moved to specialized treatment locations, rather than waiting for physicians in the wards. Stevens even went so far as to compare a good elevator to a Rolls-Royce, insisting that "service should be considered before price."[33] In the 1927 annual report of the Montreal General Hospital, L. J. Rhea, director of the Pathological Laboratory, made a direct link between elevator technology and medical progress:

> An elevator, a long hoped-for improvement, has recently been approved by our Board of Management. When this is built it will release some much needed space in the main building, as well as add greatly to the comfort of the patients, who must now climb three flights of stairs, in order that certain tests be properly made upon them. It will, in fact, make possible certain tests that we have been unable to carry out in the past.[34]

The modern hospital integrated and coordinated vast mechanized support services. The factory aesthetic and its emphasis on machinelike efficiency (no jolting and jarring) was most obvious in the more industrial sectors of the hospital, such as the service building, or in the myriad of tunnels constructed during the 1920s to connect the service sector to the patients' rooms. Like the industrial zone of the emerging modern city, the hospital service building typically accommodated messy work like the cooking, washing, and ironing, as well as housing the hospital's male and female help. "The hospital kitchen should be planned like a modern factory—that is, to receive the raw material and to deliver the finished product (which is palatable food) with as few lost motions and delays as would be expected by a modern manufacturer in his factory," wrote Stevens.[35] At the Ottawa Civic Hospital, the section (Figure 5.12) illustrates how food cars were sent through tunnels to elevators in the main building and the food was then served from ward kitchens. The ranges, steamers, deep sinks, and refrigerators were carefully arranged in the spacious main kitchen (Figure 5.13) according to studies aimed at reducing wasted steps. These recommended a single focal point, with carts traveling a minimum distance and equipment accessible from all four sides.

The new laundry (Figures 5.14 and 5.15) at the Royal Victoria Hospital, designed by Ross & Macdonald in 1931, is evidence that Stevens and Lee were not the only hospital architects concerned with isolating more industrial functions from the patients and encouraging factory-style production. Ross & Macdonald evidently agreed with the preference for strictly linear movement Stevens outlined in his book: "[A]n effort should be made to avoid lines of crossing and re-crossing; one process should follow the other until the work is complete."[36] The stark, undecorated spaces of the hospital laundry ensured that soiled linen could go smoothly from the sorting room—through the washer,

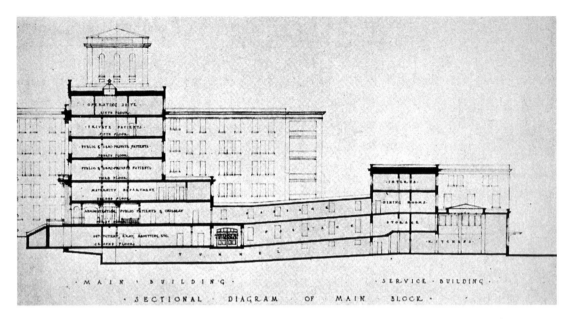

FIGURE 5.12. Section of the Ottawa Civic Hospital showing the smooth tunnel connection of the kitchen and patient rooms.

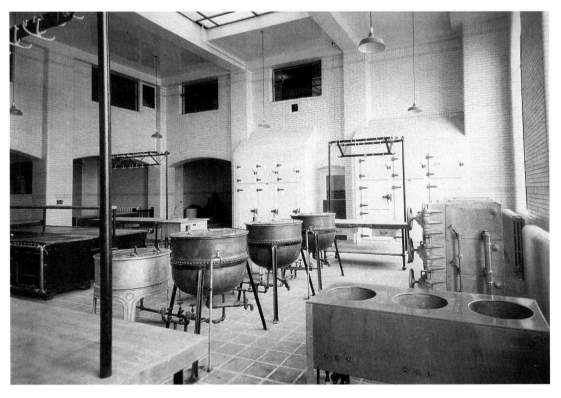

FIGURE 5.13. Architects modeled hospital kitchens after factories to maximize efficiency. Ottawa Civic Hospital kitchen, 1926.

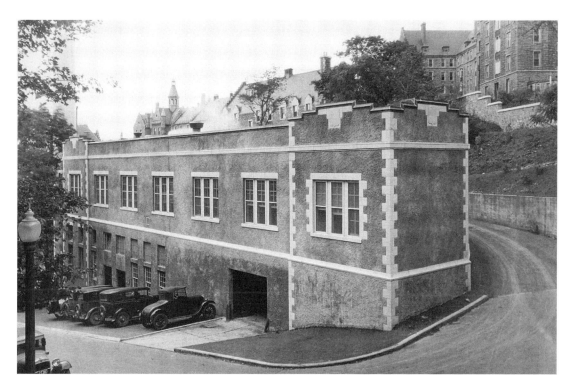

FIGURE 5.14. Exterior view, Royal Victoria Hospital laundry, 1931.

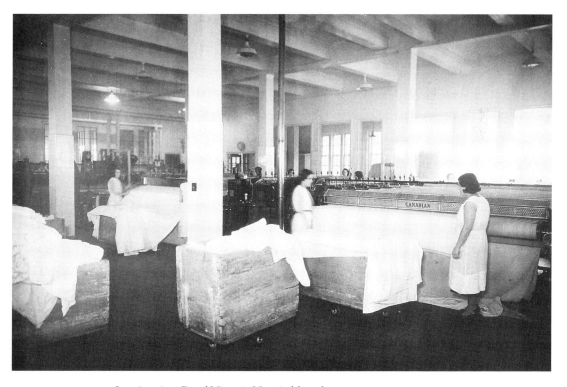

FIGURE 5.15. Interior view, Royal Victoria Hospital laundry, 1931.

extractor, flatwork ironer, drying tumbler, and steam press—to the clean linen room. This challenge for architects of the hospital laundry was related to the design problems inherent to other institutional building types, like hotels, which also tried to handle soiled materials discreetly and give (at least) the appearance of antiseptic linen.[37]

This same "image" of cleanliness informed the design of rooms occupied by patients. The emphasis on aseptic surfaces had scientific and medical implications, but also economic and ideological ones. Medical specialists developed sterilization to discourage contact (as opposed to airborne) infections. But in the interwar period it is difficult to distinguish between an overall desire for cleanliness and an attempt to stop the spread of infection. Thus even though the Pasteur Institute in France had undermined the scientific justification for the fumigation of operating and patient rooms by 1900, and C. V. Chapin's experiments in Rhode Island in 1905–8 had shown that there was no greater incidence of diphtheria and scarlet fever without fumigation, the practice continued into the 1910s.[38] The hospital had to be arranged so that disinfection could be done as efficiently as possible. Most important, these procedures could appear to have been done, which was particularly important to entice middle-class patients to accept the hospital as an institution.

The architectural counterpart to the countless cleaning products commonly used by hospitals at this time (germicide, sterilizing fluid, disposable water cups, paper towels, and various specialized soaps) was the detail that illustrated how all doors, windows, wall bases, medicine cabinets, closets, and even vents were to be located flush with the wall.[39] The floors, walls, and ceiling of the 1926 delivery room at the Ottawa Civic Hospital (Figure 5.16), for example, which appear as a continuous surface without any projecting base or trim, are typical of this trend. All the metal furniture in the room was on wheels, so that the seamless whole could be cleaned (and viewed) in a single instance. Stevens insisted on the inclusion of a covered flushing floor drain, too, in operating units so that the entire space could be hosed down.[40]

PLANS AND EXTERIORS

The rise of surgery marked a major change in hospital architecture: the transformation of the old-fashioned operating theater into the operating suite.[41] In chapter 1, we saw how older buildings featured a rather grand space in which medical students and colleagues could watch surgery performed from tiered seating. Surgery in the state-of-the-art interwar hospital took place in a much more modest setting.[42] An area of about three hundred square feet, according to Stevens, allowed the student to observe surgery from much closer up, and thus "to gain an intimate knowledge of live tissue."[43] This reduction in area also meant that more operations could be done in the same amount of space, an important parameter since surgery was in greater demand.

This increased visibility of surgery in hospital design was also perceptible from the street, as surgical suites built from about 1910 to 1940 were commonly illuminated by large windows and skylights. Skylights are, as such, a signature feature of interwar medicine. And North American hospitals tended to have multiple operating rooms, while European hospitals—even the largest ones—would have only one. Generally speaking, after World War II, electric operating lights and mechanical ventilation meant that operating rooms were often located in windowless spaces and thus became invisible from the exterior of the hospital.[44]

Historicist imagery was banned in operating suites to ensure this image of sterile, aseptic, modern medicine. But historicist decoration was clearly crucial to the image of the hospital outside of the operating room. On the exterior of the hospital service building, for example, which might be home to mundane functions such as heating, maintenance, and carpentry, it blanketed the structure's utilitarian role. And in terms of the hospital's urban image, a dignified exterior treatment expressed the dependence of hospitals on charitable donations. In the design of the original Royal Victoria Hospital by Snell in 1889–93, for example, the multiple references to Scottish baronial architecture presumably pleased the hospital's founders and administrators, many of whom had emigrated from Scotland. Stevens opted to employ this same architectural vocabulary in his two major additions to the building.

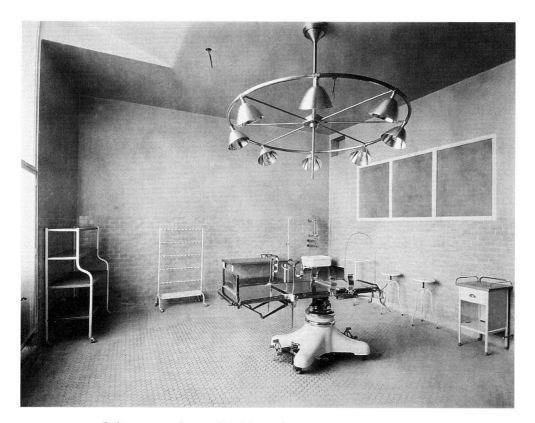

FIGURE 5.16. Delivery room, Ottawa Civic Hospital, 1926.

Stevens radically changed the theoretical basis of his professional persona by considering the exterior imagery of his hospitals of secondary importance to the plan. This is in sharp contrast to nineteenth-century architectural theorists, such as Andrew Jackson Downing, who worked hard to promote the architectural profession by arguing that building plan and exterior were inexorably if mysteriously linked.[45]

Likewise, Stevens's discussion of aesthetics in terms of the psychological impact on the viewer is much more egalitarian than the earlier emphasis on inborn taste. He frequently mentioned this "psychological effect" of the hospital's exterior in his publications, presumably in an effort to associate architecture with the new science of psychology:

> The severe, barren, forbidding exterior of the old hospital has given way to a studied architectural treatment, pleasing to the patient and the public. The small extra cost of a well designed exterior is more than repaid in its psychological effect on the entering patient and the visitor. If the patient can enter with the right impression of the institution, such impression reacts for the good of the patient's convalescence.[46]

The psychological effects of historicist decoration were especially important in the design of the hospital's administration department, which also relied on the image of the big house to conjure up comfort, trust, traditional values, and dependability. Stevens justified an ideal administration department purely in terms of psychological effects that he argued should be pursued as far as the budget would allow:

> The entrance to this department should be carefully studied from the psychological standpoint, with reference to the effect on the would-be patient. Decoration should play an important part in it. The architect should be allowed to depart from the severe design which characterizes other portions of the building, though over-elaboration should be avoided on account of its obvious expense.[47]

On the question of style, the architect pointed to the plan. In his chapter titled "Details of Construction and Finish," he explained:

> The exterior details of the hospital should be made to conform to the style of architecture in which the building is designed and should be left to the architect, it being borne in mind that the detail and exterior treatment should be subservient to the plan; in other words, the exterior should be designed around the plan, and not the plan made to suit the elevation as is so often the case.[48]

This attitude is reiterated in Stevens's published works, where he insisted, over and over again, that the test of a good hospital was its plan. He even went so far as to describe its importance in terms of a percentage. In 1915, he argued in *Architectural Record:*

Unlike most architectural problems, the plan of the hospital is the strongest factor in the design. . . . While the design should never be overlooked, the plan should hold at least eighty per cent of importance of the entire structure; and if the plan is right, we should be able to clothe it properly.[49]

The carefully orchestrated historical references made by architects like Stevens are illustrations of how hospitals responded to and encouraged social changes in health practices. The persistence of historical imagery may stem from the difficult acceptance of scientific prodecures in modern health care. Technologies at the end of the nineteenth century, like the X-ray, or at the turn of the century, like the electrocardiograph, for example, were apparently used mostly for confirmation and/or merely to satisfy physicians' curiosity (rather than as tools for diagnosis like they are today) until well after World War I. As historian of medicine Joel D. Howell has noted, "[T]he mere existence of diagnostic technology did not dictate how or where it would be used; both hospital and machine had to change before the x-ray or any other machine could significantly influence the utilization of hospital care."[50]

The white, undecorated, hard-edged architectural forms we associate with International Style architecture did not appear on the exteriors of urban general hospitals until the 1930s, and really not in full force until the 1950s. By then, there was no reason to stem the optimism for an increasingly scientific medicine. Medicine of the interwar period inspired modernist plans, but these remained embedded in historicist and classicizing exteriors that might easily have been mistaken for hotels, schools, or even town halls.

Stevens retired due to ill health in 1943. In the fall of 1940, he remarked with unusual ambivalence: "It is to be noticed that the majority of the newer large hospitals all over the world have applied the so-called modernistic architectural detail to the exterior design. This is a good sign."[51]

Coda

The use of hospital architecture as an instrument of power did not disappear with the retirement and subsequent death of Edward Stevens or even with the onset of World War II. Hospital planners today employ a similar rhetoric, based on nearly identical priorities and anxieties, to justify construction of new facilities. Echoing the way Stevens and his colleagues criticized the Victorian era of philanthropist-centered hospital building and undifferentiated wards, today's experts demonize interwar and postwar modern hospitals and even encourage their demolition.

The preservation issues surrounding hospital buildings and properties are complex. Expensive and notoriously difficult to convert, hospitals are often abandoned and fall quickly into disrepair and even ruin. Canada and the United States have seen the demolition of significant hospitals in the past decade, mostly as a result of institutional closures and mergers. Complicating the questions of reuse are thorny notions of rights and responsibility. Should public institutions become luxury housing? Hospitals such as the Royal Victoria were founded on private donations, too. Who stands to gain when the buildings become obsolete?

What we lose by converting early-twentieth-century hospitals to inappropriate new uses or demolishing them is the dignified civic presence that characterized these urban institutions. Sensitive and imaginative modernization or reuse of hospitals is possible and worthwhile. It can even augment new hospital construction, suggesting the layering of historical change that we explored in chapter 1.

Still, there are significant links between hospitals of the past and today's health-care institutions. Just as Stevens did, planners today want hospital spaces to look comforting and homelike, rather than hard-edged and high tech. Nowhere is this as evident as in the design of children's hospitals, which typically include comforting references to middle-class houses or even to child-friendly public places like zoos and trains. This arranged marriage of cozy domesticity and high technology is one of the paradoxes of postmodern architecture and a central idea behind post-1980s hospital architecture. Whereas hospitals of the 1950s and 1960s tended to look like office buildings, contemporary hospital architecture draws its inspiration from domestic architecture, hotels, and even shopping malls. Accommodation for outpatients, flexibility, efficiency, accessibility, and disguising technology and even parking remain essential features of contemporary hospital planning.

Also at issue in considering the links between past and future hospital models is a collision of architectural and medical reasoning. While architectural education frequently draws on precedents and case studies, modern medicine invests in a notion of progress that looks forward, rather than back. Hospital planners today derive much of their sense of purpose from this medical model, mistakenly presuming that new buildings necessarily lead to an improvement in medical care. Architecture and medicine thus differ in significant ways. When the fields intersect, we gain knowledge of both disciplines. When they collide, architecture is mute. Interwar experts like Stevens understood the value of studying historic precedents in order to modernize the hospital. For him, the past informed the future. My best hope is that the history of architecture will continue to enrich the future of hospitals, ensuring medicine by design.

Notes

INTRODUCTION

1. David Gagan and Rosemary Gagan report the precise growth for Ontario, Manitoba, and British Columbia in *For Patients of Moderate Means*, 3–4.

2. Perhaps because its exterior architectural messages were often conventional, the interwar hospital is generally neglected in the handful of books on the history of health-care architecture. In *The Hospital: A Social and Architectural History*, the only Western survey of hospital architecture, Thompson and Goldin jump from a discussion of the famous pavilion-plan building, Johns Hopkins in Baltimore of 1885, to skyscraper hospitals. Throughout the book is an underlying assumption that architectural innovation is a direct consequence of medical innovation, with architects acting only as deferential intermediaries.

3. The following are also useful studies of the evolution of hospital architecture: Risse, *Mending Bodies;* Sloane, "In Search of a Hospitable Hospital" and "Scientific Paragon to Hospital Mall"; Stevenson, "Medicine and Architecture."

4. Forty, "The Modern Hospital," 61.

5. Prior, "The Architecture of the Hospital," 95, 110.

6. Connor, "Bigger than a Bread Box."

7. Connor, "Hospital History." Two other useful reviews of Canadian medical history are Mitchinson, "Canadian Medical History" and "Health of Medical History."

8. The exception is Alvar Aalto's hospital at Paimio. For an extended discussion of the complexities of the terms *Modern* and *Modernism,* see Goldhagen, "Something to Talk About."

9. Social historian Mark Cortiula's work shares with this study the assumption that a detailed analysis of several institutions can allow us to generalize about a national, international, or perhaps even universal type. He also argues that the local context of a hospital is as important as the broader scientific milieu. Cortiula, "Houses of the Healers."

10. Gagan and Gagan begin their study just three years earlier, in 1890, which they see as "the beginning of the movement to reshape the public general hospital as the primary health-care centre for the whole community." Gagan and Gagan, *For Patients of Moderate Means,* 11.

11. This plan on linen is in the John Bland Canadian Architecture Collection, McGill University, dated 5 Mar. 1896.

12. Upton, *Holy Things and Profane*; Van Slyck, *Free to All* and *Manufactured Wilderness*; Cromley, *Alone Together*.

13. Fitch, *American Building*, illustration 173. The sanatorium also featured in a *Time* magazine review of modern architecture in 1944 titled "Mellowing Modernism."

14. Examples of studies that consider North American architecture include Gournay and Loeffler, "Washington and Ottawa"; Gowans, *Images of American Living*.

15. This general approach to architecture was pioneered by scholars such as Dell Upton and Paul Groth at the University of California at Berkeley. See Upton, *Holy Things and Profane*, and Groth, *Living Downtown*.

16. Pokinski, *The Development of the American Modern Style*; Solomonson, *The Chicago Tribune Tower Competition*.

17. *Official Guide and Souvenir*, 120.

18. Goulet, Hudon, and Keel, *Histoire de l'Hôpital Notre-Dame*, 47–48.

19. Lighthall, *Montreal after 250 Years*, 76.

1. 1893

1. Francophone Catholics were in the minority between the 1820s and the 1850s, but by the 1860s, they were the majority again. In 1901, the Island of Montreal was 63.9 percent French origin, 31.6 percent British origin, and 4.5 percent other origins. Francophones formed a slim majority in 1893. See Linteau, *Histoire de Montréal*, 45.

2. The notion of U, E, and H as dominant plan forms is discussed in Markus, *Buildings & Power*, 101.

3. On children's wards at the general hospital, see Adams and Theodore, "Designing for 'The Little Convalescents,'" 204–5.

4. Marsan, *Montreal in Evolution*, 257.

5. Charter of the Royal Victoria Hospital, quoted in Lewis, *Royal Victoria Hospital*, 311.

6. Lighthall, *Montreal after 250 Years*, 76.

7. Stokes, *Here and There*, 55.

8. Lighthall, *Montreal after 250 Years*, 80; Stokes, *Here and There*, 55.

9. It is difficult to find a postcard of the Royal Victoria after World War II, perhaps because its modern additions made it resemble other hospitals.

10. Notman's son William McFarlane Notman made eight trips to photograph the railway's westward journey between 1884 and 1909. He is also well known for his composite portraits. See the entries for father and son in *The Canadian Encyclopedia*, 1525–26; and Hall, Dodds, and Triggs, *The World of William Notman*, 10–11, 21–22.

11. "On the Mountain's Breast."

12. Terry, *The Royal Vic*, 177.

13. "On the Mountain's Breast."

14. *Official Guide and Souvenir*, 109.

15. The *Star* polled one hundred physicians about the proposed site in November 1888. Of the fifty-three anglophone doctors, twenty-eight thought it was too far from the city; four thought it too close to the reservoir. Of the francophones, twelve liked the site, twenty-five were against it. Of these twenty-five, fifteen thought it too far from the city, and ten opposed it on

account of the reservoir. The results are reproduced in an appendix of Howell, *Francis John Shepherd*, 233–34.

16. *Souvenir of the First Annual Convention, Master Painters' and Decorators' Association of Canada*, 73.

17. Agnew, *Canadian Hospitals*, 48–49.

18. *RVH Annual Report 1894*, 8. For the length of stays in Ontario hospitals, see Appendix J in Gagan and Gagan, *For Patients of Moderate Means*, 200.

19. Mouat published on hospital architecture and related themes independently as well. See the bibliography for samples of his interests.

20. Taylor, *The Architect and the Pavilion Hospital*, 57.

21. "Obituary." *RIBA Journal*, series 3, 11 (1904): 160.

22. Snell was also the designer of many public institutions in England, including the Boys' School for the Royal Patriotic Fund, Wandsworth, the Convalescent Home for Children, Norbiton, Holborn Union Infirmary, St. Olave's Tooly Street Union Infirmary, St. George's Hanover Square Union Infirmary, the Casual Wards, Marylebone Workhouse, the Marylebone Swimming Bath, and renovations to the Aberdeen Royal Infirmary. Snell collaborated, too, with other well-known architects. For example, he designed the Kensington Infirmary with Alfred Williams and the Dublin Exhibition with Francis Fowke. Alfred Walter Saxon Snell designed many buildings for the sick and poor. These are listed in "Obituary." *RIBA Journal* series 3, 56, no. 1 (Sept. 1949): 507. Harry is less well known, given his early death. See *Directory of British Architects 1834–1900*, 858.

23. The bequest was announced in "Mr. Saxon Snell's Bequest to the Institute."

24. "On the Mountain's Breast." The close links between physicians at the RVH and in Edinburgh are explained in Entin, "Edinburgh Medical College."

25. See my review of Jeremy Taylor's *The Architect and the Pavilion Hospital* in *Victorian Studies*. An earlier, useful study of the typology is King, "Hospital Planning."

26. A detailed overview of theories of contagion is given in Ackerknecht, "Anticontagionism."

27. Tomes, *The Gospel of Germs*, 33.

28. See Prior, "The Architecture of the Hospital," 93; Forty, "The Modern Hospital." There are also suggestions of this notion in the architectural press. See, for example, Milburn, "A Comparative Study."

29. Tomes, *The Gospel of Germs*, 8.

30. The RVH was so described in "The Royal Victoria Hospital," *Standard* (8 Aug. 1909). Royal Victoria Hospital Collection.

31. Prior, "The Architecture of the Hospital," 94–99.

32. Robson claimed in a letter to Chipman, dated 20 Apr. 1895, that thirty beds were intended, "but we have had 32 on account of the pressure." Royal Victoria Hospital Collection.

33. Snell, "Modern Hospitals," 273.

34. Undated specs for hot water heating apparatus, in the possession of the hospital, call for radiators to be covered by a Tennessee marble slab 1½ inch thick.

35. The author of "Driftwood" in 1902 also suggests that plants may have been a form of entertainment for patients: "What a boon those waving green plants are to the northern world, where more fragile plants fade and die in the heated atmosphere of our houses. Their shiny leaves allow of the daily bath of soap and water, germs of disease, and yet there is always the delight of watching the unfolding of the delicate green blades which gradually form the graceful fans

which harmonize so curiously with nearly all schemes of interior decoration." "Driftwood," *Globe*, 5 Apr. 1902. In RVH Scrapbook SCR.1 136. Royal Victoria Hospital Collection.

36. A letter from Robson to Chipman, dated 20 Apr. 1895, claims the wards are 12½ feet high and that an increase in width of 18 inches would be an improvement. Royal Victoria Hospital Collection.

37. H. Saxon Snell, "On 'Circular Hospital Wards,'" 206–7.

38. Hammond, "Reforming Architecture," 14.

39. Florence Nightingale to Henry Saxon Snell, British Library, ADD MS 45820, Folio 133–142, 17 January 1888. I am grateful to Cynthia Hammond for sending me this reference.

40. See Van Slyck, "The Lady and the Library Loafer."

41. Adams, "The Eichler Home," 169–70.

42. Milburn, "A Comparative Study," 299.

43. Wangensteen and Wangensteen, *Rise of Surgery*, 453–56.

44. I am grateful to Dell Upton for bringing my attention to this passage. Pennsylvania Hospital, Board of Managers, Minutes, vol. 9, 13 May 1833–27 Dec. 1858, Archives of Pennsylvania Hospital. Microfilm, American Philosophical Society, 24 Feb. 1845.

45. Wangensteen and Wangensteen, *Rise of Surgery*, 462.

46. I am grateful to Abigail Van Slyck for this insight.

47. Wangensteen and Wangensteen, *Rise of Surgery*, 464.

48. See, for example, Rosemary Stevens, *In Sickness and in Wealth*, 10.

49. Robson estimated the number of places differently in two separate articles about the Royal Victoria Hospital. He wrote 200 in *Hospitals, Dispensaries and Nursing*, 417, but in *Montreal Medical Journal* 22, no. 7 (Jan. 1894), 538, he claims accommodation for 250 students.

50. On elevation drawing No. 13, labeled H J K, this washroom section is crossed through in pencil and someone has written "out," perhaps indicating that these facilities were not included in the hospital as built.

51. "The Royal Victoria Hospital," *Montreal Medical Journal*, 538.

52. Boulton, "Pemberton," 452.

53. Taylor, *The Architect*, 176.

54. Ibid., 179.

55. A. Saxon Snell, "Modern Hospitals," 268.

56. Ibid., 266, 279.

57. Snell, "On 'Circular Hospital Wards,'" 209. This recommended volume of air did not change much with time. In 1925, Alfred Saxon Snell was still suggesting 1,000–1,200 cubic feet per patient. See Snell, "The Design and Equipment of Modern Hospitals," 948.

58. Snell, "On 'Circular Hospital Wards,'" 210.

59. Snell and Mouat, *Hospital Construction and Management*, 251.

60. See Snell, *Charitable and Parochial Establishments*, 21.

61. These drawings, in the John Bland Canadian Architecture Collection, render little information on the various spaces; rooms contain numbers, rather than names.

62. Lewis, *Royal Victoria Hospital*, 20.

63. Ibid.

64. Abbott to Snell, 26 March 1889. Royal Victoria Hospital Collection.

65. Howell, *Francis John Shepherd*, 233–34.

66. Adams, *Architecture in the Family Way*, 32.

67. Robson, "The Royal Victoria Hospital, Montreal," 416.

68. "Victoria Hospital, Montreal," 52.

69. Milburn, "A Comparative Study," 293.

70. The quote comes from the review of Snell and Mouat's *Hospital Construction*; see *Builder* (5 July 1884), 2.

71. Snell, "On 'Circular Hospital Wards,'" 207.

72. "The Royal Victoria Hospital," *Montreal Medical Journal* 22, no. 7 (Jan. 1894): 538.

73. Architect Andrew Taylor added the outpatients' department in 1899.

74. The hospital assembled the various documents pertaining to the fee dispute into a report titled "Memorandum Respecting Mr. Snell's letter of 22nd October 1894." Royal Victoria Hospital Collection.

75. Abbott to Stephen, 7 Feb. 1891. Royal Victoria Hospital Collection.

76. Marx, *Machine in the Garden*; both quotes are from "Social Functions," 2.

2. PATIENTS

1. "Glimpses of Some of Montreal's Hospitals," 296.

2. "Ross Pavilion," *Construction*, 191.

3. See "The Private Patient Pavilion," McGill University Archives R.G. 96 c. 329.

4. "Ross Pavilion," *Construction*, 191.

5. Ibid., 189–95.

6. "Largest Single Hospital," 25.

7. "Many Unique Features," 28; "This Telephone Switchboard," 46.

8. Macy and Bonnemaison, *Architecture and Nature*, 74, 126.

9. Stevens, *American Hospital* (1928), 101–2.

10. Ibid., 102.

11. Ibid.

12. Adams and Schlich, "Design for Control," 315.

13. Agnew, *Canadian Hospitals*, 149–78. Gagan and Gagan have shown that in 1900 in Ontario, the percentage of contributions to hospital operating incomes were almost equally shared by governments, patients, and voluntary contributions. In 1920 and 1925, patients contributed nearly 65 percent. See Gagan and Gagan, *For Patients of Moderate Means*, appendix F (1), 195.

14. See Mackintosh, *Construction, Equipment, and Management of a General Hospital*, 82–92. Mackintosh writes on p. 82: "In the out-patient department of a teaching Hospital [medical] students have an opportunity of studying the commoner ailments that they will be most frequently called upon to treat when they go into practice, but which they will never see in the wards. . . . It should also constitute part of every nurse's training, . . . more especially if she takes up district nursing among the poor."

15. "Planning Buildings for Out-patient Service," 219.

16. See Stevens, *American Hospital* (1928), 338–40.

17. Stevens included a particularly lovely photo of the waiting room for outpatients at the Ottawa Civic in the 1928 edition of *American Hospital*, 337.

18. See Stevens, *American Hospital* (1928), 322–44.

19. Gagan and Gagan, *For Patients of Moderate Means*, 172.

20. Loudon, "Childbirth," 1068.

21. Mitchinson, *Giving Birth in Canada*, 49.

22. A detailed description of the functions provided on each floor of the hospital is given in Duncan, "The Royal Victoria Montreal Maternity Hospital."

23. Barrett, "Management of the Obstetrical Department," 74–77.

24. The entry level for public patients is labeled "Tunnel level" on the drawings. Moving upward, the floors are called Sub-ground, Ground, First, Second, Third. The total number of levels and partial levels is ten. Today the entry once intended for paying patients is on the fourth floor.

25. Gagan and Gagan, *For Patients of Moderate Means*, appendix H, 198.

26. The Providence hospital is reproduced as the frontispiece in his book (and pages 187, 188, 453, and 471) and discussed at length in Stevens, "What the Past Fifteen Years Have Taught Us."

27. Stevens, "What the Past Fifteen Years Have Taught Us," 706.

28. Mitchinson, *Giving Birth in Canada*, 47–48.

29. Ibid., 164.

30. Ibid., 172–73.

31. Duncan, "The Royal Victoria Montreal Maternity Hospital," 13.

32. "Royal Victoria Maternity Hospital," *Canadian Hospital*, 14.

33. See, for example, the advertisement for Dominion Battleship linoleum in *Canadian Hospital* 3, no. 8 (Aug. 1926): 7.

34. On the significance and development of pavilion-plan hospitals, see Taylor, *The Architect and the Pavilion Hospital.* On the history of the Royal Victoria Hospital, see Lewis, *Royal Victoria Hospital.*

35. Lewis, *Royal Victoria Hospital*, 22, 26.

36. Ibid., 182. According to the late Martin Entin of the Royal Victoria Hospital, Ward N was on the third floor of Snell's east ward, facing University Street.

37. This resemblance is noted by Noah Schiff in "'The Sweetest of All Charities.'"

38. Jacalyn Duffin claims New York in 1854 was the first. See Duffin, *History of Medicine*, 317.

39. Sloane, "'Not Designed Merely to Heal,'" 332.

40. For a discussion of domestic ideology as an expression of an overtly feminist material culture, see Adams, *Architecture in the Family Way*, 158–60. On the architecture of settlement houses, see Weiner, *Architecture and Social Reform.*

41. Schiff has also noted the strategic location of the first-floor boardroom, which permitted a view of the entry from the room, while those in the boardroom remained invisible from the entry. Schiff, "'Sweetest of All Charities,'" 122.

42. Seidler, "An Historical Survey of Children's Hospitals."

43. Butler, "Planning of Children's Hospitals," 180.

44. Chapin, "Are Institutions for Infants Necessary?"

45. Stevens, *American Hospital* (1928), 210.

46. See Stevens, "Admitting Department of Buffalo Children's Hospital," which is likely his only article on children's hospitals. For a general history of the Hospital for Sick Children in Toronto, see Braithwaite, *Sick Kids.*

47. The buildings are described in "Toronto Hospital for Sick Children."

48. Stevens, *American Hospital* (1928), 218.

49. On the development of modern hospitals, see Adams, "Modernism and Medicine."

50. Goldbloom, *Small Patients*, 175–78.

51. Baker, *The Machine in the Nursery.*

52. Howell, *Technology in the Hospital.*

53. Goldbloom, *Small Patients*, 190.

54. The Shriners' Hospital is another interesting example of a children's hospital, but is outside the scope of this chapter. On its design, see "Shriners of Montreal Erecting Commodious Hospital"; and "Shriners' Hospital for Crippled Children."

55. Lemieux, *Une culture de la nostalgie*, 12.

56. These tents were probably wooden structures with canvas, pull-down walls. Four are visible in a photo of Commencement Day published in the 1912 annual report. This list of buildings has been pieced together from various sources, mostly "The Romance of a Great Idea," notes from a slide lecture given by nurse Dora Parry, probably in 1966 (Collection Montreal Children's Hospital).

57. *MCH: The Children's Story*, n.p.

58. Duffin, *History of Medicine*, 317. For a discussion of the ways in which early pediatricians justified their claim to a separate specialty, see Gillis, "Bad Habits and Pernicious Results."

59. Bensley, "Harold Beveridge Cushing," 95.

60. For biographical information on Sawyer, see "Joseph Sawyer, MRAIC: Sa personalité, son oeuvre."

61. "St. Justine's Hospital, Montreal."

62. "L'Hôpital Ste-Justine for Children."

63. Goulet, Hudon, and Keel, *Hôpital Notre-Dame de Montréal*, 108.

64. Hornstein, "Architecture of the Montreal Teaching Hospitals."

3. NURSES

1. Coburn, "'I See and Am Silent,'" 155.

2. "Kingston General Hospital," 10.

3. The other competitors were Hutchison & Wood, Taylor Hogle and Davis, Robert Findlay, Marchand and Haskell, and George A. Brown. See House Committee RVH, Minute Book 2, 1903–15, Royal Victoria Hospital Collection.

4. The architecture of nursing has been little explored by historians; the most thorough study is Kingsley, "The Architecture of Nursing." On the Royal Victoria Hospital Training School in particular, see Catterill, *The Alumnae Association Incorporated;* deForest, *Proud Heritage;* and Munroe, *The Training School for Nurses.* The school closed in 1972, although the association is still active. A longer history of nursing education at the Montreal General Hospital, an English-speaking hospital founded in 1819, is offered in MacDermot, *History of the School for Nurses of the Montreal General Hospital.* The histories of francophone nursing education at Montreal hospitals are found in Daigle, "Devenir infirmière." On the history of training schools in Canada, see Gibbon and Mathewson, *Three Centuries of Canadian Nursing.*

5. McPherson, *Bedside Matters*, 31.

6. MacDermot, *History of the School for Nurses of the Montreal General Hospital*, 51.

7. Excerpted from the Royal Victoria Hospital's Act of Incorporation, Charter of the Royal Victoria Hospital, Statutes of Canada, 50–51 Victoria (1887), chapter 125, reproduced in Lewis, *Royal Victoria Hospital,* 311–15. The main responsibilities of a new probationer at the hospital in 1894 are listed in Gibbon and Mathewson, *Three Centuries of Canadian Nursing,* 159.

8. Lewis, *Royal Victoria Hospital,* 26.

9. Ibid., 128. The Royal Infirmary at Edinburgh, the model for the Royal Victoria Hospital, had a separate dining room for nurses designed by David Bryce.

10. It became the doctors' dining room after construction of the Maxwells' residence for nurses and stood until the construction of the new surgical wing in 1955. Confusingly, the 1905 plans show a different space labeled "dining room" in the western end of the administration building; this was likely the servants' dining room.

11. "On the Mountain's Breast," col. 1–2. Other plans sometimes indicate spaces in the medical and surgical wings, such as the notation "Head Nurse" on an unenclosed space in the East ventilation tower (1905 plans); the function of these spaces, however, seems to have changed fairly frequently. Nurses at the nearby Montreal General Hospital slept in "cubicles built into an old ward, and after a stormy night, their beds were often festooned with snow." This quotation is cited in Coburn, "'I See and am Silent,'" 136.

12. Lewis, *Royal Victoria Hospital,* 135.

13. The instructional aspects of mid-twentieth-century nurses' residences are mentioned in Townley, "The Planning of Nurses' Homes." Examples are illustrated in "Burton Hall Women's College Hospital Residence," "Student Nurses' Residence," and "Royal Alexandra Nurses Residence." The nurses' home constructed at the Montreal General Hospital in 1926 also contained "a complete teaching unit of laboratories and class rooms, all on one floor." See MacDermot, *History of the School for Nurses of the Montreal General Hospital,* 65.

14. Note that the 1905 plans have a space labeled "classroom" among the nurses' bedrooms on the fourth floor. The hospital-based training of nurses in Canada was gradually replaced by college and university programs, beginning in 1920 at the University of British Columbia. See Coburn, "'I See and Am Silent,'" 153, and Stewart, *It's Up to You,* 31–42. Stewart has noted that the establishment of this pioneering program satisfied a need on the part of hospital administrators to create a hierarchy within nursing, rather than reflecting a sincere interest on the part of the university to welcome women. For more information on the history of nursing in Quebec, see Cohen and Dagenais, "Le métier d'infirmière"; and Daigle, Rousseau, and Saillant, "Des traces sur la neige."

15. *1933 Yearbook,* 19. Royal Victoria Hospital Collection.

16. Nineteenth-century medical advice literature written for women, for example, is full of suggestions that menstruation, conception, and even childbirth would be eased by rural or natural surroundings. See Adams, *Architecture in the Family Way,* 104.

17. On ideologies of women and nature informing the process of suburbanization, see Wright, *Moralism and the Model Home;* and Adams, "The Eichler Home."

18. These prestigious structures included the first pathology building and medical theater (1894), the new pathology building by Nobbs & Hyde (1924), and the Montreal Neurological Institute by Ross & Macdonald (1933–34).

19. The Royal Victoria Hospital has never owned property east of University; it has always belonged to the Royal Institute for the Advancement of Learning (McGill University). The possibility remains that the nurses' home was constructed west of the hospital because of legal

issues restricting the medical buildings on the site. There are few references to the siting of build-ings in the hospital's documents; the Board of Governors' Minute Book (23 September 1902) notes, however, that Andrew Taylor's design for a new surgical theater extension at right angles to the surgical wing (that is, onto the land leased from the city) was rejected partly due to concern about building on city property. Royal Victoria Hospital Collection.

20. Eileen C. Flanagan, "An Address Given at the 75th Reunion Royal Victoria Hospital Nurses' Alumnae." 9 May 1972, 7. Royal Victoria Hospital Collection.

21. Kingsley has remarked that many nurses' residences had doors of exceptional architectural merit, which lent the institution "identity and stature" and also marked the transition between work and home. Kingsley, "The Architecture of Nursing," 78. This door at the Royal Victoria Hospital, however, was an interior door from the hospital. Royal Victoria Hospital nurses were often photographed at the entry to the Lawson & Little extension.

22. Gibbon and Mathewson, *Three Centuries of Canadian Nursing*, 376.

23. Stevens, *American Hospital* (1928), 403; Thomas Harris, on the other hand, writing twenty-five years earlier, remarked that most nursing homes adjoined general hospitals. See Harris, "Notes on a Short Visit," 114.

24. Stevens, *American Hospital* (1928), 403.

25. Photographs of these social spaces intended as enticements to the profession appear throughout the promotional literature. See the pamphlet *So You Want To Be A Nurse?* Royal Victoria Hospital Collection.

26. MacLennan, "The New Residence," 18–19.

27. On apartments for women, see Cromley, *Alone Together*, 112–15; and Pearson, *Architecture and Social History of Cooperative Living*, 45–55. The relationship of British apartment buildings for women to Victorian feminism is analyzed in Adams, *Architecture in the Family Way*, 152–58.

28. For an analysis of the complex, multifunctional Grey Nuns' motherhouse, see Martin, "Housing the Grey Nuns." For a comparison of the Hôtel-Dieu (a convent-hospital) and the Royal Victoria Hospital in terms of medical space, see Hornstein, "Architecture of the Montreal Teaching Hospitals." Kingsley cites monasteries and military hospitals as important precedents for nurses' buildings; see Kingsley, "Architecture of Nursing," 65–66.

29. See Miller, "The Big Ladies' Hotel." On women's colleges in general, see Horowitz, *Alma Mater.*

30. It is interesting to note that the Maxwells were involved in additions or alterations to at least three Canadian buildings by Price: the Chateau Frontenac (1919–24), Windsor Station (1899–1901), and the James Ross house (1897–98).

31. See House Committee RVH, Minutes Book 2, 1903–15, Royal Victoria Hospital Collec-tion. Separate quarters for nurses were also included in a list of suggestions made by the Med-ical Board following the fire of 1905. See Lewis, *Royal Victoria Hospital*, 135. Lord Strathcona is mainly remembered as a financier of the Canadian Pacific Railroad. He was also chief commissioner of the Hudson's Bay Company, a member of Parliament, president of the Bank of Montreal, and Canadian High Commissioner to the United Kingdom.

32. Vicinus, *Independent Women*, 129; the book includes a chapter on reformed nursing (85–120).

33. Comments on the uniform are taken from a letter from Miss Janet Marlane to a friend, reprinted in the *1925 Yearbook*, Royal Victoria Hospital Collection. Coburn, "'I See and Am Silent,'" 135–40.

34. Stevens, *American Hospital* (1928), 406.

35. See "House of H. Vincent Meredith."

36. The house is now referred to as the Lady Meredith House; when Lady Meredith bequeathed the house to the Royal Victoria Hospital in 1940 or 1941, it became the Joint Hospital Institute of Montreal. The Charles Meredith House next door became a residence for Royal Victoria Hospital nurses after 1941. Edward S. Clouston's house on Peel Street was also designed by the Maxwells (1893–94) and used for a nurses' residence; he was Royal Victoria Hospital president from 1910 to 1912. See Lewis, *Royal Victoria Hospital*, 236; Rémillard and Merrett, *Montreal Architecture*, 147, 172.

37. George Weir's *Survey of Nursing Education in Canada* of 1932 emphasized the role of the dietetic lab in nursing education so that nurses could become "ambassadors to the people of the new preventive medicine." Gibbon and Mathewson, *Three Centuries of Canadian Nursing*, 376.

38. *1933 Yearbook*, 19, Royal Victoria Hospital Collection. Stevens illustrated the plans of fifteen nurses' residences, many of which include educational spaces, in his chapter on the building type. See Stevens, *American Hospital* (1928), 403–39. Some large hospitals even had separate educational facilities for nurses at this time. See ibid., 437–39, especially his Figure 523, the model plan of an educational building for nurses as suggested by the New York State Board of Nurse Examiners. The Royal Victoria Montreal Maternity Hospital included housing for its nurses on its sixth floor, with a demonstration room, living room, and library. See ibid., 193.

39. Mrs. Daley applied to Sir Donald A. Smith for admission to the school. The House Committee Minute Book documents that "as it appeared that Mrs. Daley was married and at present living with her husband it was decided that it would not be advisable to accept her application." See House Committee RVH, Minute Book, 1893–1903 (12 June 1895), 98, Royal Victoria Hospital Collection.

40. Eileen C. Flanagan, "An Address Given at the 75th Reunion Royal Victoria Hospital Nurses' Alumnae." 9 May 1972, 7. Royal Victoria Hospital Collection.

41. *1933 Yearbook*, 19, Royal Victoria Hospital Collection.

42. Telephone interview with Lynda deForest, 31 March 1994. She is a graduate of the Royal Victoria Hospital training school and the author of a history of the school (*Proud Heritage*).

43. This innovative design was featured in a photograph of a double room in the *1933 Yearbook*, 19. Royal Victoria Hospital Collection.

44. Eileen C. Flanagan, "An Address Given at the 75th Reunion Royal Victoria Hospital Nurses' Alumnae," 9 May 1972, 2. Royal Victoria Hospital Collection. Flanagan was elected president of the Alumnae Association in 1939. The changes carried out during her term are outlined in the Alumnae Association booklet.

45. Such advertisements are the subject of Adams, "Building Barriers."

46. Eileen C. Flanagan, "An Address Given at the 75th Reunion Royal Victoria Hospital Nurses' Alumnae," 9 May 1972, 1, 2. Royal Victoria Hospital Collection. Goodhue was president of the Alumnae Association from 1913 to 1923.

47. Hersey's obituary by Elsie Allder appeared in *Canadian Nurse* 101 (Feb. 1949): 3. Some of her accomplishments are cited in Gibbon and Mathewson, *Three Centuries of Canadian Nursing*, 172–73.

48. Lewis, *Royal Victoria Hospital*, 135; the possibility exists, of course, that the Lady Superintendent resided in the first nurses' home despite the suggestions of the Medical Board and the lack of indications on the plan; alternatively, she may have received rooms in the 1917 expansion.

49. After the 1905 fire, the Board of Governors decided the superintendent should live on-site.

Lodging for him and his family was built on the western end of the administration building (Lewis, *Royal Victoria Hospital*, 135). According to his obituary in *Canadian Hospital* 3, no. 12 (Dec. 1926), 29, the hospital's second superintendent, Henry Edward Webster, died at his hospital residence.

50. Lewis, *Royal Victoria Hospital*, 249.

51. The housemen received their first billiard room in the 1898 extension to the administration block designed by Andrew Taylor (Lewis, *Royal Victoria Hospital*, 128). The other social spaces provided in 1930 included a generous lounge; the second and third floors had a living room and sitting room, respectively. The plans of the interns' building were published in Parry, "Review of the Recent Exhibition of Hospital Architecture," 425.

4. ARCHITECTS AND DOCTORS

1. Bartine, "The Building of the Hospital Departments and Rooms," 263.

2. Letter from Elizabeth Andrews, reference archivist, Massachusetts Institute of Technology, 10 Feb. 1995.

3. Boston of Today, 1892, typewritten page sent from the Boston Public Library. There is no record of Stevens's employment at McKim, Mead & White, however, in the firm's archives in the Avery Architectural and Fine Arts Library at Columbia University (letter from Janet Parks, curator of drawings, Columbia University, New York, dated 19 July 1995). Next to nothing is known of his personal life, except that he married twice (was widowed in 1905) and had one daughter, whose name is listed inconsistently in sources. Stevens belonged to a number of conservative groups, through which he may have made important hospital contacts. He was a Republican, a Mason, an Episcopalian (another source says Congregationalist), and a member of the University and City clubs in Boston. He was a member of the American Institute of Architects, the Royal Architectural Institute of Canada, the Province of Quebec Association of Architects, and the American Hospital Association.

4. See "Some Recent Hospitals." Some buildings of Kendall, Taylor & Company are listed in Bertrand E. Taylor's entry in Withey, *Biographical Dictionary of American Architects*. He died in 1909. See also the entry for Henry H. Kendall, who died in 1943.

5. Stevens, "The Transformation of a Dwelling House," in *Modern Hospital*, and same title, in *The Architect and Engineer of California*.

6. In 1912, Brown recounted their impressions in two pieces for *Hospital World*, both titled "European Hospital Notes." On his career, see Henry J. Morgan, ed., *The Canadian Men and Women of the Time: A Handbook of Canadian Biography of Living Characters* (Toronto: William Briggs, 1912), 155; and Connor, *Doing Good*, 175, 302.

7. Stevens, "The Contagious Hospital," 183–84.

8. See Brown and Stevens, "A General Hospital for One Hundred Patients," and Brown, "European Hospital Notes," 166.

9. Stevens frequently noted the lack of provisions for various therapies in American hospitals by showing slides of European examples. See Stevens, "The Need of Better Hospital Equipment for the Medical Man," 253–88.

10. A list of Stevens's journal articles is included in the bibliography.

11. "The American Hospital of the Twentieth Century," 128.

12. These partners were George A. Curtin, Herbert G. Mason, and William A. Riley.

13. "Activities of the Institute."

14. Fleury, "Hospital Planning."

15. York & Sawyer founded their partnership in 1898 and are best known for their design of large banks and hospitals, including the Rockefeller and Fifth Avenue hospitals, Corning Hospital, Hospital for Special Surgery, and Lenox Hill Hospital in New York, Mountainside Hospital, Glen Ridge, N.J., Rhode Island Hospital Trust Co., Providence, Saint Paul's Hospital in Manila, Children's Hospital and Allegheny General Hospital, in Pittsburgh, Wilmington General Hospital, Wilmington, Del. See "York and Sawyer" in *Macmillan Encyclopedia of Architects* (1982), 460–61. Like Stevens, York and Sawyer worked as young architects for McKim, Mead, & White; and like Lee, Sawyer studied at the École des Beaux-Arts in Paris.

16. Gournay, "Gigantism," 174.

17. Stevens's addition to the Detroit hospital was published in Edward F. Stevens, "The Surgical Unit," 18.

18. The formation of their partnership was announced in *Hospital World* in an article titled "Canada."

19. The biographical information on Lee is scanty. See *Who's Who in Canada* (1925–26), 179–80. Lee was the author of at least two journal articles. "Planning the Construction" had first been presented at the convention of the Ontario Hospital Association in Toronto, 1–3 Oct. 1930.

20. *Hospital World* described the Toronto General Hospital in "The New Toronto General Hospital," although the architects are unnamed. Lee alone signed the ground floor plan reproduced in Hollobon, *The Lion's Tale*, 17.

21. This number is mentioned in several obituaries. See "E. F. Stevens, Architect, Dies in 86th Year," *Boston Herald*, 1 Mar. 1946, 33; "Edward F. Stevens, Noted Architect, 85," *New York Times*, 1 Mar. 1946, 22; "Obituary," *Modern Hospital* 66, no. 4 (Apr. 1946): 176. Stevens appears in several biographical sources, notably *National Cyclopaedia of American Biography* (1927), B: 244–45; *Who Was Who in America* (1942–51), 2:509; and *Who's Who in America* (1940–41), 2460. Note that Stevens's entry in Withey contains several major errors.

A list of Stevens and Lee's most significant Canadian buildings includes the additions to the Royal Victoria Hospital, Montreal; the Ottawa Civic Hospital; Hôpital Notre-Dame, Montreal; Kingston General; Moncton City Hospital, Moncton, New Brunswick; Brandon, Manitoba; Women's College Hospital, Wellesley Hospital, St. Joseph's Hospital, the Connaught Laboratories, I.O.D.E. Preventorium, and the 1912 Hospital for Sick Children, Toronto; parts of Victoria General Hospital and Halifax Children's Hospital; Hôtel-Dieu de Saint-Sacrement in Quebec; St. Joseph's Hospital in Guelph, Hamilton, and Peterborough, Ontario. The firm acted as consultants on the Brantford General Hospital, the Pathological Building at McGill/Royal Victoria Hospital, and the Metropolitan General Hospital, Walkerville, Ontario, among others.

Stevens and Lee's best-known American hospitals were the General Hospital at New Britain, Conn.; Lying-in Hospital, Providence, R.I.; General Hospital in Buffalo, N.Y.; Barre City Hospital, Barre, Vt.; St. Luke's Hospital in Jacksonville, Fla.; the Springfield (or City) Hospital in Springfield, Mass.; and the Ohio Valley General Hospital, in Wheeling, W.Va. They also designed Sea View Hospital, Staten Island, N.Y.; the Central New England Sanatorium, Rutland, Mass.; Lawrence Memorial Hospital, Medford, Mass.; Lawrence General Hospital, Lawrence, Mass.; and Worcester City Hospital, Worcester, Mass. In addition, the firm did a series of hospitals (Police, Mixto, Obrero, Maternidad) in Lima, Peru.

22. I am grateful to David Theodore for this calculation. He determined that of 15,412 hospital beds available in 1935 in Canada, 5,105 (or 33 percent) were in Stevens and Lee–designed buildings. Similarly, of 551 interns in Canadian hospitals in 1935, 193 (or 35 percent) were in Stevens and Lee buildings. The list of hospitals he used appears in "Approved General Hospitals," 446.

23. *National Cyclopaedia of American Biography*, 245.

24. See "Awards Made," 43.

25. "Well Known Hospital Architects Form Partnership," 29; "The Federal Government Discontinues Hospital Advisory Service," *Canadian Medical Association Journal* 27, no. 5 (Nov. 1932): 55; see "Obituary," *Journal (Royal Architectural Institute of Canada)* 19, no. 2 (Feb. 1942): 35. A list of Parry's publications is included in the bibliography.

26. "Obituary," *Journal (Royal Architectural Institute of Canada)* 19, no. 2 (Feb. 1942): 35.

27. Smith, "Planning a General Hospital," 13.

28. Smith to Chenoweth, 12 May 1932. Royal Victoria Hospital Collection.

29. Ibid.

30. Ibid.

31. See "A Point or Two on Hospital Planning"; "Regarding Hospital Planning"; Goodnow, "Importance of Detail" and "The Utility Room."

32. "Regarding Hospital Planning."

33. Stevens, *American Hospital* (1918), 247.

34. After the war, wounded men were given all these products free of charge, "instead of having to pay the almost prohibitive prices charged before the war." See Robert D. Defries, "The War Work of the Connaught," 96. Insulin was also produced there; in fact, the Connaught Laboratories were described as "the largest insulin factory in the world." See Edwards, "A Peacetime Munitions Plant," 63.

35. A description of the Connaught Laboratories is "New Laboratories of Toronto University"; see also Fitzgerald, "The War-Work of the Connaught and Antitoxin Laboratories."

36. On Eden Smith, see Adams, "Eden Smith." On Nobbs, see Wagg, *Percy Erskine Nobbs.*

37. A description of the process is in "Anti-Toxin for Canadian Soldiers."

38. Gooderham was also responsible for choosing Stevens and Lee as architects. The process by which they were hired and the property chosen is spelled out in a letter and historical narrative, likely written by John G. Fitzgerald to Robert Falconer, 8 Oct. 1935. J. G. FitzGerald, Historical Memo, October 1935, Sanofi Pasteur Limited (Connaught Campus) Archives, 83-001-09. I am grateful to Christopher Rutty for bringing this material to my attention.

39. Defries, "The War Work of the Connaught," 96.

40. "New Laboratories of Toronto University," 881.

41. Stevens, "Qualifications of the Hospital Architect."

42. Schlereth, *Victorian America*, 65–66.

43. See Burdett's remarks following Bartine, "The Building of the Hospital Departments and Rooms," 285.

44. Ibid.

45. Stevens, *In Sickness and in Wealth*, 156–58.

46. Gournay, *Ernest Cormier*, note 24. Goldwater's ideas were collected posthumously in a 1947 book titled *On Hospitals*. For a list of his articles from 1905 to 1942, see its bibliography, 385–92.

47. Walsh and Martin, "Hospital Planning," 286.

48. Ibid., 286–87.

49. On the general role of water in medicine, see Porter, ed., *Medical History of Water and Spas.*

50. Brown and Stevens, "A General Hospital for One Hundred Persons," 136–37.

51. Stevens's paper was published twice within months of the conference under the title "The Need of Better Hospital Equipment for the Medical Man" in *Modern Hospital* and *Hospital World.* The stormy reception of his ideas is suggested in a report on his paper; see "Urges Elaborate Hospitals," 227–28.

52. Stevens, "The Physiotherapy Department of the American Hospital," 18. This text repeats in chapter 6 of *American Hospital* (1928), 160.

53. See Gritzer and Arluke, *The Making of Rehabilitation,* 58; Larkin, "The Emergence of Para-Medical Professions," 1333.

54. Stevens, *American Hospital* (1928), 164.

55. Ibid., 151, 152, 154, 155.

56. See "Natural Daylight Not Suited to Operating Room Requirements."

57. See Adams and Schlich, "Design for Control."

58. A general history of the OCH is *"Fisher's Folly."*

59. For more information on the buildings, see "A Three and a Half Million Dollar Hospital"; and Stevens, "How Ottawa Is Solving Its Hospitalization Problem."

60. "Exteriorization of Urban Hospitals," 181.

61. Stevens, *In Sickness and in Wealth,* 69.

62. Unsigned copy of a letter to Sir Vincent Meredith, 5 Aug. 1919. City of Ottawa Archives, Ottawa Civic Hospital, Box 61, "Reports," Civic Hospital Committee 1919–27.

63. Bower, report read before the Civic Hospital Board, 30 Aug. 1919. City of Ottawa Archives, Box 61, "Reports," Civic Hospital Committee 1919–27. The description is from a memorandum attached to the report, dated 15 Sept. 1919.

64. Stevens, *American Hospital* (1921), 8.

65. Stevens to Robertson, 12 Mar. 1920. City of Ottawa Archives M638 Box 62, "Stevens & Lee."

66. A list of other hospital architects following this model would include Allen B. Pond and Irving K. Pond. There seem to have been no female architects who specialized in hospital design prior to World War II.

5. MODERNISMS

1. "Notre Dame Hospital, Montreal, Completes $1,500,000 Building Program," 17.

2. More research is needed to determine the geographic extent of these trends. Some hospitals in Europe in the 1920s also combined traditional exteriors and modern planning. I am grateful to Adrian Forty and Christine Stevenson for pointing to the Middlesex Hospital in London as an interesting parallel to the work of Stevens and Lee. Designed by Alner W. Hall in 1927–35, the new building was built in phases. Its H-plan included modern features: medical and surgical wards, separate space for women, four large operating theaters. Middlesex Hospital is red brick and Portland stone, supported by a steel frame. It is described in Richardson, *English Hospitals,* 37–38, as "a still fashionable neo-Georgian, perhaps with a few transatlantic overtones." For a history of the institution, see Saunders, *The Middlesex Hospital.* On the influence of many American institutions, excluding hospitals, on European architecture, see Cohen, *Scenes of the World to Come.*

3. "Notre Dame Hospital, Montreal, Completes $1,500,000 Building Program," 17, 26.

4. See "The Hospital and the Community It Serves," 17–19.

5. Stevens, *American Hospital* (1928), 5–6.

6. See "Preparing the Trays."

7. Agnew, "The Reduction of Noise in Hospitals," 24.

8. Boyce, "Noise," 199.

9. Stevens used Celotex in the corridors of the Ross Pavilion at the Royal Victoria Hospital; see Lindahl, "Relieving the Noise Evil in Hospitals," 36.

10. A copy of this detail, dated Aug. 20, 1925, is in the Archives of Ontario, Arthur Heeney Jr. Collection, C-27, series D.

11. "Hospital Noises and How to Minimize Them." For more on Stevens's ideas about sound control, also see the article he published titled "Sound Absorption, Insulation and Air Control."

12. An interesting discussion of the apparent flexibility (related to increased occupation) of a hospital of all-private rooms is found in Thompson and Goldin, *The Hospital*, 207–25.

13. Ford, *My Life and Work*, 216. Ford's perspective is particularly relevant since he founded, paid for, and built a hospital in 1915.

14. Stevens, *American Hospital* (1928), 42.

15. Stevens, "The Open Ward vs. Single Rooms," 233. Thompson and Goldin have noted how the trend toward private accommodation was completely obliterated by the Depression, as almost instantly nobody at all could afford private rooms and hospitals remodeled them as semiprivate. See Thompson and Goldin, *The Hospital*, 216.

16. "Montreal Jewish General Hospital Opens with Impressive Ceremony."

17. On the history of linoleum, see Simpson, "Linoleum and Lincrusta."

18. The supplier of rubber to the Royal Victoria Hospital in 1926, Gutta Percha & Rubber, Ltd., of Toronto, expressed considerable hesitation in this specification, stating that the plans for rubber on the walls and ceiling were "something quite beyond our sphere." See letter from J. H. S. Kerr to H. E. Webster, 10 May 1926. Royal Victoria Hospital Collection.

19. Smith, "Development and Planning," 370. The subject of flooring was often discussed in the professional literature. Stevens's ideas on hospital floors were articulated in "More about Hospital Floors" and "A Discussion of Hospital Floors"; and later in "The Trend in Hospital Construction," 31–32.

20. "Ross Pavilion," *Construction*, 191; a contemporary comparison of a hotel and hospital lobby is found in Pearson, "Some Modern American Hospitals," 643.

21. Stevens, *American Hospital* (1928), 28.

22. "A Heated Garage for Hospital Doctors."

23. Morman, *Efficiency, Scientific Management, and Hospital Standardization*, n.p. [11].

24. These statistics are from MacEachern, "What Is Hospital Standardization?" 8. On standardization in general, see Morman, *Efficiency, Scientific Management, and Hospital Standardization*; Stephenson, "The College's Role"; Stevens, *In Sickness and in Wealth*, 105–39.

25. Examples of these include "Introduction to the Architectural Check Lists"; *Hospital Yearbook 14*: entire issue.

26. See "Introduction to the Architectural Check Lists." Goldwater's obituary stated that he was also a registered architect and an "advisory construction expert for 156 hospitals in the United

States, Canada, Newfoundland and British Columbia." See "Dr. S. S. Goldwater is Dead Here at 69." *New York Times,* 23 Oct. 1942, 21.

27. This "negotiation of cognitive exclusiveness" as essential to the development of specialist professions is explained by sociologist Magali Larson in *The Rise of Professionalism,* 15–18, 30–31. For a discussion of how architects developed professional authority along these lines, see Upton, *Architecture in the United States,* 247–83.

28. Stevens, "How Ottawa Is Solving Its Hospitalization Problem," 69.

29. Stevens, "The Trend in Hospital Construction," 24.

30. "Last Word in Hospital Design," 486. The plan in *American Hospital* (1928), 94, shows sixteen-bed wards, partitioned into groups of four.

31. Howell, *Technology in the Hospital,* 30–68. On the impact of Taylorism and scientific management in general, see Giedion, *Mechanization Takes Command,* 77–127.

32. Stevens, *American Hospital* (1928), 497.

33. "Construction Section," 369–70.

34. *Montreal General Hospital 106th Annual Report,* 72.

35. Stevens, *American Hospital* (1928), 443.

36. Ibid., 468.

37. On the hotel laundry, see "A Modern Hotel Laundry." The sanitary reform of hotels, Pullman cars, and restaurants is included in Tomes, *The Gospel of Germs,* 172–82.

38. Richardson, "The Fetish of Fumigation" and "Should Private Rooms Be Disinfected?"

39. See Pite, "Hospital Operating Theatres."

40. Stevens, "The Surgical Unit," 20.

41. Note that Stevens's design for Notre-Dame included a small teaching amphitheater, typical of his teaching hospitals. In 1932 he referred to the amphitheater operating room as "almost a thing of the past except in intensive teaching hospitals." See Stevens, "The Trend in Hospital Construction," 26. His ideas on operating rooms were articulated in his articles on the subject. See Stevens, "The Surgical Unit"; Foss and Stevens, "An Ideal Operating Suite."

42. An account of the disappearance of the surgical amphitheater is given in Wangensteen and Wangensteen, *The Rise of Surgery,* 453–73.

43. Stevens, *American Hospital* (1928), 140.

44. For more on the history of daylight in operating theaters, see chapter 1. Stevens stated as early as 1932 that "the old skylight is rarely seen" and that artificial illumination was generally preferred to daylight. Windows, however, were still used for ventilation. See Stevens, "The Trend in Hospital Construction," 26.

45. See Downing, *Architecture of Country Houses.*

46. Stevens, "The Trend in Hospital Construction," 24.

47. Stevens, *American Hospital* (1928), 27. Stevens suggested that hospitals should reflect their surroundings (i.e., that suburban hospitals should appear more domestic), while urban hospitals should be more "stately." See Stevens, "What the Past Fifteen Years Have Taught Us," 705.

48. Stevens, *American Hospital* (1928), 493.

49. Stevens, "The American Hospital Development, Part II," 645.

50. Howell, "Machines and Medicine," 132.

51. Stevens, "Newer Trends in Hospital Plans and Equipment," 83.

Bibliography

Unarchived manuscript sources (such as letters, minute books, yearbooks) appear only in the notes, including the institution in which they were found (e.g., Royal Victoria Hospital Collection). Archival sources, obituaries, and reference works also appear only in notes with full reference information.

Ackerknecht, Erwin H. "Anticontagionism between 1821 and 1867." *Bulletin of the History of Medicine* 22 (1948): 562–93.

"Activities of the Institute." *Journal (Royal Architectural Institute of Canada)* (Sept. 1929): 347.

Adams, Annmarie. *Architecture in the Family Way: Doctors, Houses, and Women, 1870–1900.* Montreal: McGill-Queen's University Press, 1996.

———. "Building Barriers: Images of Women in the RAIC Journal, 1924–73." *Resources for Feminist Research* 23, no. 3 (Fall 1994): 11–23.

———. "Eden Smith and the Canadian Domestic Revival." *Urban History Review* 21, no. 2 (Mar. 1993): 104–15.

———. "The Eichler Home: Intention and Experience in Postwar Suburbia." In *Perspectives in Vernacular Architecture.* Vol. 5, *Gender, Class, and Shelter,* edited by Elizabeth Collins Cromley and Carter L. Hudgins, 164–78. Knoxville: University of Tennessee Press, 1995.

———. "Modernism and Medicine: The Hospitals of Stevens and Lee, 1916–1932." *Journal of the Society of Architectural Historians* 58, no. 1 (Mar. 1999): 42–61.

———. "Of Monuments and Men: A Review of *Montréal Métropole.*" *Canadian Historical Review* (Sept. 1999): 473–79.

———. Review of *The Architect and the Pavilion Hospital,* by Jeremy Taylor. *Victorian Studies* 41, no. 3 (Spring 1998): 550–53.

———. Review of *Doing Good: The Life of Toronto's General Hospital,* by J. T. H. Connor, and *The Provincial Asylum in Toronto: Reflections on Social and Architectural History,* by Edna Hudson, ed. *Canadian Historical Review* 83, no. 1 (Mar. 2002): 110–14.

———. Review of *Healthcare Architecture in an Era of Radical Transformation,* by Stephen Verderber and David J. Fine. *Journal of the Society of Architectural Historians* 59, no. 4 (Dec. 2000): 556–57.

———. "Rooms of Their Own: The Nurses' Residences at Montreal's Royal Victoria Hospital." *Material History Review* 40 (Fall 1994): 29–41.

———, and Thomas Schlich. "Design for Control: Surgery, Science, and Space at the Royal Victoria Hospital, Montreal, 1893–1956." *Medical History* 50, no. 3 (July 2006): 303–24.

———, and David Theodore. "Designing for 'The Little Convalescents': Children's Hospitals in Toronto and Montreal, 1875–2006." *Canadian Bulletin of Medical History* 19, no. 1 (2002): 201–43.

Agnew, G. Harvey. *Canadian Hospitals, 1920–1970: A Dramatic Half Century.* Toronto: University of Toronto Press, 1974.

———. "The Reduction of Noise in Hospitals." *Canadian Hospital Annual Reference Book* 8 (Jan. 1931): 23–26.

Aikens, Charlotte, ed. *Hospital Management.* Philadelphia: W. B. Saunders, 1911.

"The American Hospital of the Twentieth Century." *Hospital World* 14, no. 4 (Oct. 1918): 127–28.

"Anti-Toxin for Canadian Soldiers All Made at Toronto University." *Toronto Star Weekly,* 25 Nov. 1916.

"Approved General Hospitals." *Canadian Medical Association Journal* 32, no. 4 (1935): 446.

"Awards Made in the Recent Exhibition of the Toronto Chapter Ontario Association of Architects." *Journal (Royal Architectural Institute of Canada)* (26 Feb. 1926): 43.

Baker, Jeffrey P. *The Machine in the Nursery: Incubator Technology and the Origins of Newborn Intensive Care.* Baltimore: The Johns Hopkins University Press, 1996.

Barrett, Caroline V. "Management of the Obstetrical Department." *Bulletin of the AHA* 6, no. 1 (Jan. 1932): 74–77.

Bartine, Oliver H. "The Building of the Hospital Departments and Rooms." *Transactions of the AHA* 18 (1916): 262–87.

Bensley, Edward H. "Harold Beveridge Cushing (1873–1947)." In *McGill Medical Luminaries,* 95–97. Montreal: Osler Library, 1990.

Boulton, Marilyn E. "The Pemberton Memorial Operating Room 1896–1925: Part I." *BC Medical Journal* 27, no. 7 (July 1985): 450–502.

Boyce, H. A. "Noise." *Canadian Nurse* 6, no. 5 (May 1910): 196–200.

Braithwaite, Max. *Sick Kids: The Story of the Hospital for Sick Children in Toronto.* Toronto: McClelland and Stewart, 1974.

Brandt, Allan, and David C. Sloane. "Of Beds and Benches: Building the Modern American Hospital." In *The Architecture of Science,* edited by Peter Galison and Elizabeth Thomson, 281–308. Cambridge, Mass.: MIT Press, 1999.

Brown, John N. Elliott. "European Hospital Notes." *Hospital World* 1, no. 3 (Mar. 1912): 166–72; (Apr. 1912): 244–64.

———, and Edward Fletcher Stevens. "A General Hospital for One Hundred Patients." In *Hospital Management,* edited by Charlotte Aikens, 108–47. Philadelphia: Saunders, 1911.

"Burton Hall Women's College Hospital Residence and School of Nursing." *Journal (Royal Architectural Institute of Canada)* 33 (Apr. 1956): 124.

Butler, Charles. "Planning of Children's Hospitals." *Brickbuilder* 19, no. 8 (Aug. 1910): 180–86.

———, and Addison Erdman. *Hospital Planning.* New York: F. W. Dodge, 1946.

"Canada." *Hospital World* 1, no. 3 (1912): 210.

Catterill, Kathryn. *The Alumnae Association Incorporated of the Royal Victoria Hospital Training School for Nurses 1896–1972.* Montreal: RVH, 1972.

Chapin, Henry Dwight. "Are Institutions for Infants Necessary?" *Journal of the American Medical Association* 64 (2 Jan. 1915): 1–3.

Coburn, Judi. "'I See and Am Silent': A Short History of Nursing in Ontario." In *Women at Work, Ontario, 1850–1930,* edited by Janice Acton, Penny Goldsmith, and Bonnie Shepard, 127–63. Toronto: Canadian Women's Educational Press, 1974.

Cohen, Jean-Louis. *Scenes of the World to Come: European Architecture and the American Challenge.* Paris: Flammarion; Montreal: Canadian Centre for Architecture, 1995.

Cohen, Yolande, and Michèle Dagenais. "Le métier d'infirmière: Savoirs féminins et reconnaissance professionnelle." *Revue d'histoire de l'amerique française* 41, no. 2 (Fall 1987): 155–77.

"Connaught Laboratories, University of Toronto." *Construction* 99 (May 1918): 153–56.

Connor, J. T. H. "Bigger than a Bread Box: Medical Buildings as Museum Artifacts." *Caduceus* 4, no. 2 (Autumn 1993): 119–30.

———. *Doing Good: The Life of the Toronto General Hospital.* Toronto: University of Toronto Press, 2000.

———. "Hospital History in Canada and the United States." *Canadian Bulletin of Medical History* 7 (1990): 93–104.

"Construction Section." *Transactions of the American Hospital Association* 29 (1927): 367–72.

Copp, Terry. "Public Health in Montreal, 1870–1930." In *Medicine in Canadian Society: Historical Perspectives,* edited by S. E. D. Shortt, 395–415. Montreal: McGill-Queen's University Press, 1981.

Cortiula, Mark William. "Houses of the Healers: The Changing Nature of General Hospital Architecture in Hamilton, 1850–1914." *Histoire Sociale/Social History* 28, no. 55 (May 1995): 27–50.

Cromley, Elizabeth Collins. *Alone Together: A History of New York's Early Apartments.* Ithaca, N.Y.: Cornell University Press, 1990.

Daigle, Johanne. "Devenir infirmière: Les systemes d'apprentissage et la formation professionnelle à l'Hôtel-Dieu de Montréal, 1920–1970." Ph.D. diss., Université du Québec à Montréal, 1990.

———, Nicole Rousseau, and Francine Saillant. "Des traces sur la neige: La contribution des infirmières au développement des régions isolées du Québec au XXe siècle." *Recherches féministes* 6, no. 1 (1993): 93–103.

deForest, Lynda. *Proud Heritage: A History of the Royal Victoria Hospital Training School for Nurses, 1894–1972.* Montreal: Alumnae Association of the RVH, 1994.

Defries, Robert D. "The War Work of the Connaught and Antitoxin Laboratories, University of Toronto." *Varsity Magazine Supplement* (1918): 94–96.

Downing, A. J. *The Architecture of Country Houses.* 1850. Reprint, New York: Dover, 1969.

Duffin, Jacalyn. *History of Medicine: A Scandalously Short Introduction.* Toronto: University of Toronto Press, 1999.

Duncan, J. W. "The Royal Victoria Montreal Maternity Hospital." *Queen Charlotte's Quarterly* (Apr. 1932): 13–19.

Edwards, Frederick. "A Peacetime Munitions Plant." *Maclean's* 41, no. 2 (15 Jan. 1928): 3–5, 59, 62, 63.

Entin, M. A. "Edinburgh Medical College at the End of the Eighteenth Century and the Training of North American Doctors." *Proceedings of the Royal College of Physicians Edinburgh* (1998): 28, 218–28.

"Exteriorization of Urban Hospitals." *Hospital, Medical and Nursing World* 26, no. 6 (Dec. 1924): 181–82.

"Fisher's Folly": A History of the Ottawa Civic Hospital 1924–1984. Brochure published by the hospital to celebrate its sixtieth anniversary, 1984.

Fitch, James Marston. *American Building: The Forces That Shape It.* Boston: Houghton, Mifflin, 1947.

Fitzgerald, J. G. "The War Work of the Connaught and Antitoxin Laboratories, University of Toronto." *Varsity Magazine Supplement* (1917): 54–55.

Fleury, W. E. "Hospital Planning." *Journal (Royal Architectural Institute of Canada)* (May 1948): 182.

Ford, Henry, in collaboration with Samuel Crowther. *My Life and Work.* London: Heinemann, 1923.

Forty, Adrian. "The Modern Hospital in France and England." In *Buildings and Society: Essays on the Social Development of the Built Environment,* edited by Anthony King, 61–93. London: Routledge and Kegan Paul, 1980.

Foss, Harold L., and Edward F. Stevens. "An Ideal Operating Suite." *Modern Hospital* 44, no. 2 (Feb. 1935): 65–69.

Gagan, David. *"A Necessity Among Us": The Owen Sound General and Marine Hospital 1891–1985.* Toronto: Published for Grey Bruce Regional Health Centre by University of Toronto Press, 1990.

———, and Rosemary Gagan. *For Patients of Moderate Means: A Social History of the Voluntary Public General Hospital in Canada, 1890–1950.* Montreal: McGill-Queen's University Press, 2002.

Gibbon, John Murray, and Mary S. Mathewson. *Three Centuries of Canadian Nursing.* Toronto: Macmillan, 1947.

Giedion, Siegfried. *Mechanization Takes Command: A Contribution to Anonymous History.* New York: Norton, 1948.

Gillis, Jonathan. "Bad Habits and Pernicious Results: Thumb Sucking and the Discipline of Late-Nineteenth-Century Paediatrics." *Medical History* 40, no. 1 (Jan. 1996): 55–73.

"Glimpses of Some of Montreal's Hospitals." *Modern Hospital* 15, no. 4 (Oct. 1920): 296–305.

Goldbloom, Alton. *Small Patients: The Autobiography of a Children's Doctor.* Toronto: Longmans, 1959.

Goldhagen, Sarah Williams. "Something to Talk About: Modernism, Discourse, Style." *Journal of the Society of Architectural Historians* 64, no. 2 (June 2005): 144–67.

Goldwater, Sigismund Schulz. "Basic Ideas in Hospital Planning." *Modern Hospital* 16, no. 4 (Apr. 1921): 305–9.

———. "Hospital Construction: 1918 and After." *Modern Hospital* 12 (1919): 4–6.

———. "Hospital Planning and Construction in 1922." *Modern Hospital* 20, no. 1 (Jan. 1923): 1–4.

———. *On Hospitals.* New York: Macmillan, 1947.

Goodnow, Minnie. "Importance of Detail in Hospital Planning." *International Hospital Record* 15, no. 11 (July 1912): 10–12.

———. "The Utility Room." *International Hospital Record* 15, no. 12 (Aug. 1912): 14–16.

Goulet, Denis, François Hudon, and Othmar Keel. *Histoire de l'Hôpital Notre-Dame de Montréal, 1880–1980.* Montreal: VLB, 1993.

Gournay, Isabelle, ed. *Ernest Cormier and the Université de Montréal.* Montreal: CCA, 1990.

———. "Gigantism in Downtown Montreal." In *Montreal Metropolis, 1880–1930,* edited by Isabelle Gournay and France Vanlaethem, 153–82. Montreal: CCA, 1998.

———, and Jane C. Loeffler. "Washington and Ottawa: A Tale of Two Embassies." *Journal of the Society of Architectural Historians* 61 (Dec. 2002): 480–507.

Gowans, Alan. *Images of American Living: Four Centuries of Architecture and Furniture as Cultural Expression.* Philadelphia: Lippincott, 1964.

Gréber, Jacques. *L'architecture aux États-Unis.* Paris: Payot, 1920.

Gritzer, Glenn, and Arnold Arluke. *The Making of Rehabilitation: A Political Economy of Medical Special-ization, 1890–1980.* Berkeley and Los Angeles: University of California Press, 1985.

Groth, Paul Erling. *Living Downtown: The History of Residential Hotels in the United States.* Berkeley and Los Angeles: University of California Press, 1994.

Hall, Roger, Gordon Dodds, and Stanley Triggs. *The World of William Notman.* Toronto: McClelland and Stewart, 1993.

Hammond, Cynthia. "Reforming Architecture, Defending Empire: Florence Nightingale and the Pavilion Hospital." *Studies in the Social Sciences: (Un)healthy Interiors; Contestations at the Intersection of Public Health and Private Space* (July 2005): 1–24.

Harris, Thomas. "Notes on a Short Visit to Some of the Hospitals and Medical Educational Institutions in the United States and Canada." *Montreal Medical Journal* 32, no. 2 (1903): 109–20.

"A Heated Garage for Hospital Doctors." *Canadian Medical Association Journal* 22, no. 1 (Jan. 1930): 108–9.

Hollobon, Joan. *The Lion's Tale: A History of the Wellesley Hospital, 1912–1987.* Toronto: Irwin, 1987.

"L'Hôpital Ste-Justine for Children, Montreal, Earns Splendid Reputation." *Canadian Hospital* 5, no. 10 (Oct. 1928): 20–21.

Hornstein, Shelley. "The Architecture of the Montreal Teaching Hospitals of the Nineteenth Century." *Journal of Canadian Art History* 14, no. 1 (1991): 12–24.

Horowitz, Helen Lefkowitz. *Alma Mater: Design and Experience in the Women's Colleges from the Nineteenth-Century Beginnings to the 1930s.* New York: Knopf, 1984.

"The Hospital and the Community It Serves." *Modern Hospital Year Book* 1 (1919): 13–38.

"Hospital Noises and How to Minimize Them." *Modern Hospital* 24 (June 1925): 511.

"House of H. Vincent Meredith, Montréal." *Canadian Architect and Builder* 9 (Jan. 1896): 2.

Howell, Joel D. "Machines and Medicine: Technology Transforms the American Hospital." In *The American General Hospital: Communities and Social Contexts,* edited by D. E. Long and J. Goldin, 109–34. Ithaca, N.Y.: Cornell University Press, 1989.

———. *Technology in the Hospital: Transforming Patient Care in the Early Twentieth Century.* Baltimore: The Johns Hopkins University Press, 1995.

Howell, William Boyman. *Francis John Shepherd, Surgeon: His Life and Times.* Toronto: Dent, 1934.

"Introduction to the Architectural Check Lists." In *The Hospital Yearbook* 13, 1–2. Chicago: Modern Hospital Publishing, 1934.

"Joseph Sawyer, MRAIC: Sa personalité, son oeuvre." *Architecture-Bâtiment-Construction* 8 (janvier 1953): 19–21, 34.

Kane, Josephine. *The History of the Hospital for Sick Children, College Street, Toronto, Ont., Canada, and the Lakeside Home for Little Children, Summer Branch of the Hospital, Toronto Island.* Toronto: [Evening Telegram], 1918.

King, Anthony. "Hospital Planning: Revised Thoughts on the Origin of the Pavilion Principle in England." *Medical History* 10 (1966): 360–73.

Kingsley, Karen. "The Architecture of Nursing." In *Images of Nurses: Perspectives from History, Art, and Literature,* edited by Anne Hudson Jones, 63–94. Philadelphia: University of Pennsylvania Press, 1988.

"Kingston General Hospital Completes Its Re-Construction Scheme." *Canadian Hospital* 8, no. 5 (May 1931): 10–12.

"The Largest Single Hospital, Medical, Educational Unit on the Continent." *Canadian Hospital* 7, no. 5 (May 1930): 25–27.

Larkin, Gerald. "The Emergence of Para-Medical Professions." In *Companion Encyclopedia of the History of Medicine,* edited by W. F. Bynum and Roy Porter, 2:1329–49. London: Routledge, 1993.

Larson, Magali Sarfatti. *The Rise of Professionalism: A Sociological Analysis.* Berkeley and Los Angeles: University of California Press, 1977.

"The Last Word in Hospital Design." *Contract Record and Engineering Review* 38 (21 May 1924): 486.

Lee, Frederick. "Planning the Construction of the Small Model Hospital." In *Canadian Hospital Annual Reference Book,* 8 (Jan. 1931): 9–11.

———. "The Notre Dame Hospital, Montreal, P.Q." *Construction* 15, no. 4 (Apr. 1922): 105–9.

"Lee, Frederick Clare." *Who's Who in Canada 1925–1926,* 179–80. Toronto: International Press, 1926.

Lemieux, Denise. *Une culture de la nostalgie: L'enfant dans le roman québecois de des origins à nos jours.* Montreal: Boréal, 1984.

Lewis, David Sclater. *Royal Victoria Hospital 1887–1947.* Montreal: McGill University Press, 1969.

Lighthall, W. D. *Montreal after 250 Years.* Montreal: Grafton, 1892.

Lindahl, R. L. "Relieving the Noise Evil in Hospitals." *Canadian Hospital Annual Reference Number* 9, no. 1 (Jan. 1932): 34–37.

Linteau, Paul-André. *Histoire de Montréal depuis la Confédération.* Montreal: Boréal, 1992.

Loudon, Irvine S. L. *A Bibliography of Canadian Medical Periodicals, with Annotations.* Montreal: Renouf, 1934.

———. "Childbirth." In *Companion Encyclopedia of the History of Medicine,* edited by W. F. Bynum and Roy Porter, 2:1050–71. London: Routledge, 1993.

———. *History of the School of Nursing of the Montreal General Hospital.* Montreal: Alumnae Association, 1940.

MacDermot, H. E. *History of the School for Nurses of the Montreal General Hospital.* Montreal: Alumnae Association, 1940.

MacEachern, M. T. "What Is Hospital Standardization?" *McGill News* 3 (Sept. 1922): 7–8.

Mackintosh, Donald James. *Construction, Equipment, and Management of a General Hospital.* Edinburgh: W. Hodge, 1909.

MacLennan, E. A. E. "The New Residence." *1933 Yearbook* [Royal Victoria Training School for Nurses], 18–19.

Macy, Christine, and Sarah Bonnemaison. *Architecture and Nature: Creating the American Landscape.* London: Routledge, 2003.

"Many Unique Features Are Incorporated in New Private Patients Pavilion." *Canadian Hospital* 7, no. 5 (May 1930): 28–32, 38.

Markus, Thomas A. *Buildings and Power: Freedom and Control in the Origin of Modern Building Types.* London: Routledge, 1993.

Marsan, Jean-Claude. *Montreal in Evolution.* Montreal: McGill-Queen's University Press, 1981.

Martin, Tania. "Housing the Grey Nuns: Religion and Women in Fin-de-siècle Montréal." M.Arch. thesis, McGill University, 1995.

Marx, Leo. *The Machine in the Garden: Technology and the Pastoral Ideal in America.* New York: Oxford University Press, 1981.

MCH: The Children's Story, n.p. Brochure published to celebrate the Montreal Children's Hospital's fiftieth anniversary.

McPherson, Kathryn. *Bedside Matters: The Transformation of Canadian Nursing, 1900–1992.* Toronto: Oxford University Press, 1996.

"Mellowing Modernism." *Time,* 21 Aug. 1944, 44.

Milburn, William. "A Comparative Study of Modern English, Continental, and American Hospital Construction." *RIBA Journal*, 3rd ser., 20 (1913): 281–305.

Miller, Deborah. "'The Big Ladies' Hotel': Gender, Residence, and Middle-Class Montreal: A Contextual Analysis of the Royal Victoria College, 1899–1931." M.Arch. thesis, McGill University, 1998.

Mitchinson, Wendy. "Canadian Medical History: Diagnosis and Prognosis." *Acadiensis* 12, no. 1 (1982): 125–35.

———. *Giving Birth in Canada 1900–1950.* Toronto: University of Toronto Press, 2002.

———. "Health of Medical History." *Acadiensis* 20, no. 1 (1990): 253–64.

"A Modern Hotel Laundry." *Canadian Hotel Review* 5 (Nov. 1927): 13–14.

"Montreal Jewish General Hospital Opens with Impressive Ceremony." *Canadian Hospital* 11, no. 11 (Nov. 1934): 5.

"More about Hospital Floors." *International Hospital Record* 18 (Dec. 1914): 9.

Morman, Edward T., ed. *Efficiency, Scientific Management, and Hospital Standardization: An Anthology of Sources.* New York: Taylor & Francis, 1989.

Mouat, Frederic J. "Classification of Hospitals." *Lancet* ii (3 Sept. 1881): 408–10; (24 Sept. 1881): 536–38.

———. "Conclusion." *Lancet* ii (1 Oct. 1881): 580–81.

———. "The Construction and Arrangement of Hospitals." *Lancet* i (18 June 1881): 979–82; (25 June 1881): 1017–19.

———. "The Control and Management of Hospitals." *Lancet* i (11 June 1881): 942–44.

———. "The General Hospital of Friedrickshain in Berlin." *Lancet* ii (23 July 1881): 125–27.

———. "Hospital of St. Eloi at Montpellier, France." *Lancet* ii (9 July 1881): 41–43.

———. "Menilmontant." *Lancet* ii (2 July 1881): 3–5.

———. "On Hospitals: Their Management, Construction, and Arrangements in Relation to the Successful Treatment of Disease, with Remarks on the Organisation of Medical Relief in the Metropolis. General Introduction." *Lancet* i (4 June 1881): 902–3.

———. "Organization of Medical Relief in the Metropolis." *Lancet* ii (16 July 1881): 78–82.

"Mr. Saxon Snell's Bequest to the Institute." *RIBA Journal*, 3rd ser., 11 (6 Feb. 1904): 174.

Munroe, Marjorie Dobie. *The Training School for Nurses, Royal Victoria Hospital, 1894–1943.* Montreal: Gazette Printing, 1943.

Murray, Irena, ed. *Edward & W. S. Maxwell: A Guide to the Archive.* Montreal: CAC, 1986.

"Natural Daylight Not Suited to Operating Room Requirements." *Canadian Hospital* 7, no. 2 (Feb. 1930): 36–37.

"New Laboratories of Toronto University." *Contract Record*, 24 (October 1917): 881–83.

"New Ottawa Civic." *Construction* 13 (Dec. 1920): 370–74.

"The New Toronto General Hospital." *Hospital World* 4 (July 1913): 36–45.

"Notre Dame Hospital, Montreal, Completes $1,500,000 Building Program." *Canadian Hospital* 9, no. 6 (June 1932): 12–17, 26.

Official Guide and Souvenir: British Medical Association Sixty-fifth Annual Meeting, Montreal, 1897. Montreal: Desbarats, 1897.

"On the Mountain's Breast." *Gazette* (Montreal), 12 Nov. 1891, 2.

Parry, B. Evan. "The Administration Unit in the General Hospital." *Journal (Royal Architectural Institute of Canada)* 14 (Oct. 1937): 209–11.

———. "An Analysis of the Complexities of Hospital Construction." *Canadian Hospital* 11, no. 5 (May 1934): 10–16, 32–34; 11, no. 6 (June 1934): 5–8, 26.

———. "The Clearing House of the Modern Hospital World." *Canadian Hospital* 10, no. 4 (Apr. 1933): 9–10, 34; 10, no. 5 (May 1933): 3–5.

———. "The Economics of Hospital Planning." *Canadian Hospital* 9, no. 9 (Sept. 1932): 9–10, 25.

———. "General Problems of Hospital Construction." *Canadian Hospital* 10, no. 1 (Jan. 1933): 7–8, 26; 10, no. 2 (February 1933): 11–12, 21; 10, no. 3 (March 1933): 5–6, 24.

———. "Hospital Construction of the Twentieth Century." *Canadian Hospital* 9, no. 8 (Aug. 1932): 14.

———. "The Hospital of Yesterday and Tomorrow." *Canadian Hospital* 14, no. 11 (Nov. 1937): 13–14.

———. "Hospitals—Their Planning and Equipment." *Journal (Royal Architectural Institute of Canada)* 7, no. 6 (June 1930): 220–30; 7, no. 8 (Aug. 1930): 299–309; 8, no. 1 (Jan. 1931): 23–33.

———. "The International Hospital Congress and Annual Convention of the American Hospital Association." *Journal (Royal Architectural Institute of Canada)* 6 (Sept. 1929): 310–13.

———. "The Modern Trend of Hospital Architecture in Europe." *Canadian Hospital* 13, no. 3 (Mar. 1936): 29–32.

———. "The Modernization of a Hospital." *Canadian Hospital* 12, no. 1 (Jan. 1935): 6–7.

———. "The New Deal for Hospital Construction." *Canadian Hospital* 11, no. 3 (Mar. 1934): 4–5, 25.

———. "New Developments in Hospital Construction and Equipment." *Canadian Hospital* 12, no. 3 (Mar. 1935): 24–25, 28.

———. "Pertinent Notes on Hospital Planning and Construction." *Canadian Medical Association Journal* 21, no. 5 (Nov. 1929): 599–600.

———. "Progress versus Obsolescence." *Canadian Hospital* 11, no. 11 (Nov. 1934): 11–12, 26.

———. "The Report of the Sub-Committee of the Canadian Hospital Council on General Problems of Construction and Equipment." *Canadian Hospital* 9, no. 12 (Dec. 1932): 8–9, 26–27.

———. "Review of the Recent Exhibition of Hospital Architecture Held in Toronto." *Journal (Royal Architectural Institute of Canada)* (Dec. 1931): 423–27.

———. "Sweden Leads the Way." *Canadian Hospital* 14, no. 3 (Mar. 1937): 34–35.

"Pathology's Scope Needs Broadening Says Dr. Boycott." *Gazette* (Montreal), 7 Oct. 1924, 8.

Pearson, Lionel G. "Recent Developments in Hospital Planning Abroad." *RIBA Journal*, 3rd ser., 34 (1926–27): 503–22.

———. "Some Modern American Hospitals." *Architects' Journal*, 28 Oct. 1925, 643.

Pearson, Lynn F. *The Architectural and Social History of Cooperative Living.* London: Macmillan, 1988.

Pite, William A. "Hospital Operating Theatres." *Architects' Journal*, 24 June 1925, 972.

"Planning Buildings for Out-patient Service: General Principles." *Modern Hospital* (Mar. 1926): 219.

"A Point or Two on Hospital Planning." *International Hospital Record* 17, no. 33 (27 Mar. 1914): 10–11.

Pokinski, Deborah Frances. *The Development of the American Modern Style.* Ann Arbor, Mich.: UMI Research Press, 1984.

Porter, Roy, ed. *The Medical History of Water and Spas.* Medical History, Suppl. no. 10. London: Wellcome, 1990.

"Preparing the Trays." *International Hospital Record* (15 Sept. 1914): 10.

Prior, Lindsay. "The Architecture of the Hospital: A Study of Spatial Organization and Medical Knowledge." *British Journal of Sociology* 39, no. 1 (1988): 86–113.

"Regarding Hospital Planning." *International Hospital Record* 17, no. 18 (29 Oct. 1913): 5.

Rémillard, François, and Brian Merrett. *Montreal Architecture: A Guide to Styles and Buildings.* Translated by Pierre Miville-Deschênes. Montreal: Meridian Press, 1990.

Review of *Hospital Construction and Management,* by F. J. Mouat and H. Saxon Snell. *Builder* 67 (5 July 1884): 1–2.

Richardson, D. L. "The Fetish of Fumigation—A Relic of the Past." *Modern Hospital* 33 (Aug. 1929): 90–91.

———. "Should Private Rooms Be Disinfected after Patients with Simple Infections Have Left Them?" *International Hospital Record* (25 Sept. 1914): 8.

Richardson, Harriet, ed. *English Hospitals 1660–1948: A Survey of Their Architecture and Design.* Swindon, England: Royal Commission on the Historical Monuments of England, 1998.

Risse, Guenter, B. *Mending Bodies, Saving Souls: A History of Hospitals.* New York: Oxford University Press, 1999.

Robson, Jno. J. "The Royal Victoria Hospital, Montreal." In *Hospitals, Dispensaries and Nursing,* edited by John S. Billings and Henry M. Hurd, 415–17. Baltimore: The Johns Hopkins Press, 1894.

"Ross Pavilion of the Royal Victoria Hospital." *Construction* 10 (June 1917): 189–95.

"Ross Pavilion of the Royal Victoria Hospital, Montreal." *Modern Hospital* 12, no. 5 (May 1919): 311–15.

"Royal Alexandra Nurses Residence and School of Nursing." *Journal (Royal Architectural Institute of Canada)* (Jan. 1962): 48.

"The Royal Victoria Hospital." *Canada Medical and Surgical Journal* 15 (May 1887): 625.

"Royal Victoria Hospital." *Medical Journal and Engineering Record* (17 Apr. 1929): 468–9.

"The Royal Victoria Hospital." *Montreal Medical Journal* 17 no. 1 (July 1888): 72–3.

"The Royal Victoria Hospital." *Montreal Medical Journal* 22, no. 6 (Dec. 1893): 478.

"The Royal Victoria Hospital." *Montreal Medical Journal* 22, no. 7 (Jan. 1894): 534–55.

"The Royal Victoria Hospital." *Montreal Medical Journal* 25, no. 3 (Sept. 1896): 282.

"Royal Victoria Hospital Montreal: The Modernization Program." *Journal (Royal Architectural Institute of Canada)* (Nov. 1959): 385–88.

"Royal Victoria Hospital, Montreal." *Builder* 54 (14 Jan. 1888): 34; 65 (1 July 1893): 18–19.

"Royal Victoria Hospital, Montreal." *Lancet* ii (29 Aug. 1896): 612.

"The Royal Victoria Maternity Hospital." *Canadian Hospital* 3, no. 10 (Oct. 1926): 11–15.

Saunders, Hilary St. George. *The Middlesex Hospital 1745–1948.* London: M. Parrish, 1949.

Schiff, Noah. "'The Sweetest of All Charities': The Toronto Hospital for Sick Children's Medical and Public Appeal, 1875–1905." M.A. Thesis, University of Toronto, 1999.

Schlereth, Thomas J. *Victorian America: Transformations in Everyday Life, 1876–1915.* New York: HarperCollins, 1991.

Seidler, Edward. "An Historical Survey of Children's Hospitals." In *The Hospital in History,* edited by Lindsay Granshaw and Roy Porter, 181–97. London: Routledge, 1989.

"Shriners' Hospital for Crippled Children, Montreal." *Journal (Royal Architectural Institute of Canada)* (July 1927): 242–49.

"The Shriners of Montreal Erecting Commodious Hospital for Crippled Children." *Contract Record and Engineering Review,* 28 May 1924, 540.

Simpson, Pamela H. "Linoleum and Lincrusta: The Democratic Coverings for Walls and Floors." In *Perspectives in Vernacular Architecture*. Vol. 7, *Exploring Everyday Landscapes,* edited by Annmarie Adams and Sally McMurry, 281–92. Knoxville: University of Tennessee Press, 1997.

Sloane, David Charles. "In Search of a Hospitable Hospital." *Dartmouth Medicine* (Fall 1993): 23–31.

———. "'Not Designed Merely to Heal': Progressive Reformers and Children's Hospitals." *Journal of the Gilded Age and Progressive Era* 4, no. 4 (October 2005): 331–54.

———. "Scientific Paragon to Hospital Mall: The Evolving Design of the Hospital, 1885–1994." *Journal of Architectural Education* 48, no. 2 (Nov. 1994): 82–98.

Smith, Harold J. "The Development and Planning of a Large General Hospital." *Construction* (Dec. 1924): 361–74.

———. "Planning a General Hospital." *Canadian Hospital* 2, no. 4 (1925): 13–15.

Snell, Alfred Walter Saxon. "The Design and Equipment of Modern Hospitals." *Architects' Journal,* 24 June 1925, 946–51.

———. "Modern Hospitals." *RIBA Journal,* 3rd ser., 20 (1913): 265–80.

Snell, H. Saxon. *Charitable and Parochial Establishments.* London: B. T. Batsford, 1881.

———. "On 'Circular Hospital Wards.'" In *Transactions of the Sanitary Institute of Great Britain,* 205–14. London: Sanitary Institute, 1888.

———, and Frederic J. Mouat. *Hospital Construction and Management.* London: Churchill, 1883.

"Social Functions." *Montreal Daily Star,* 2 Sept. 1897, 2.

Solomonson, Katherine. *The Chicago Tribune Tower Competition: Skyscraper Design and Cultural Change in the 1920s.* Chicago: University of Chicago Press, 2001.

"Some Recent Hospitals by Kendall, Taylor & Co." *Architectural Record* 41 (Mar. 1917): 231–53.

Souvenir of the First Annual Convention, Master Painters' and Decorators' Association of Canada. Montreal: n.p., 1904.

Stephenson, George W. "The College's Role in Hospital Standardization." *Bulletin of the American College of Surgeons* (Feb. 1981): 17–29.

Stevens, Edward Fletcher. "Admitting Department of Buffalo Children's Hospital." *Modern Hospital* 24, no. 4 (Apr. 1925): 346.

———. "The American Hospital Development, Part I." *Architectural Record* 38 (Dec. 1915): 641–61; "American Hospital Development, Part II." *Architectural Record* 39, no. 1 (Jan. 1916): 65–83.

———. *The American Hospital of the Twentieth Century.* New York: Architectural Record, 1918. Rev. ed., New York: Architectural Record Co., 1921; 2nd rev. ed. New York: F. W. Dodge, 1928.

———. "Architecture and Equipment of the Barre City Hospital." *Modern Hospital* 5, no. 5 (Nov. 1915): 338–40.

———. "Can Hospital Equipment Be Standardized?" *Modern Hospital* 13, no. 4 (Oct. 1919): 287–89.

———. "The Contagious Hospital." *Brickbuilder* 17, no. 9 (Sept. 1908): 183–84.

———. "Details of Planning General Hospitals." *Architectural Forum* 37, no. 6 (Dec. 1922): 263–70.

———. "Development of the Hospital Ward Unit of the United States Army." *Modern Hospital* 12, no. 6 (June 1919): 408–16.

———. "A Discussion of Hospital Floors." *International Hospital Record* (15 Sept. 1914): 5–6.

———. "The Fundamental Principles of the Planning, Construction and Fittings of Central Laboratories in Larger Hospitals." *Nosokomeion* 7, no. 3 (July 1936): 205–11.

———. "The Home for Nurses." *National Hospital Record* (June 15, 1908): 4–5.

———. "Hospital Noises and How to Minimize Them." *Modern Hospital* 24, no. 6 (June 1925): 511–13.

———. "How Ottawa Is Solving Its Hospitalization Problem." *Modern Hospital* 26, no. 1 (Jan. 1926): 69–72.

———. "How to Make Modern the Old Well Built Hospital." *Modern Hospital* 40, no. 3 (Mar. 1933): 45–47.

———. "The Medical School Hospital." *Architectural Record* 60, no. 2 (Aug. 1926): 112–28.

———. "Memorial Hall of Buffalo General Hospital." *Modern Hospital* 11, no. 1 (July 1918): 20–33.

———, et al. *Modern Hospitals: A Series of Authoritative Articles on Planning Details and Equipment, as Exemplified by the Best Practice in this Country and Europe.* New York: American Architect, 1912.

———. "Modernization of Nurses' Home Need Not Be Costly." *Modern Hospital* 42, no. 4 (Apr. 1934): 45–48.

———."Modernizing the Old Hospital." *Modern Hospital* 24, no. 3 (Mar. 1925): 219–24.

———. "The Need of Better Hospital Equipment for the Medical Man." *Hospital World* 6, [sic] no. 6 (Dec. 1914): 253–58.

———. "The Need of Better Hospital Equipment for the Medical Man." *Modern Hospital* 3, no. 6 (Dec. 1914): 367–71.

———. "Newer Trends in Hospital Plans and Equipment." *Hospitals* 14 (Oct. 1940): 83–84.

———. "The Nurses' Residence." *Modern Hospital* 18, no. 4 (Apr. 1922): 322–24.

———. "The Open Ward vs. Single Rooms." *Modern Hospital* 18, no. 3 (Mar. 1922): 233–34.

———. "Ottawa Pools Her Hospitals." *Modern Hospital* 15, no. 5 (Nov. 1920): 344–48.

———. "Our War Hospitals in France." *Architectural Record* 43, no. 3 (Mar. 1918): 257–84.

———. "The Physiotherapy Department of the American Hospital." *Architectural Record* 60, no. 1 (July 1926): 18–24.

———. "Planning a Fifty Bed Hospital for Beauty as Well as Utility." *Modern Hospital* 30, no. 2 (Feb. 1928): 63–64.

———. "The Planning of the Small Hospital." *Modern Hospital* 19, no. 6 (Dec. 1922): 497–502.

———. "Qualifications of the Hospital Architect." *Journal of the A.I.A.* 4, no. 5 (Oct. 1945): 169–71.

———. "The Room of the Sick in the Hospital." *Nosokomeion* 8, no. 2 (Apr. 1937): 136–37.

———. "A Sanatorium for the Well-to-do." *Modern Hospital* 17, no. 5 (Nov. 1921): 391–92.

———. "A Small Community Hospital." *Journal of the AMA* 74, no. 18 (1 May 1920): 1273–74.

———. "Small Hospitals." *Journal of the AMA* 84, no. 13 (28 Mar. 1925): 952–60.

———. "Some Construction Problems in Planning the Small Hospital." *Modern Hospital* 28, no. 3 (Mar. 1927): 100–103.

———. "Sound Absorption, Insulation and Air Conditioning of the Modern Hospital." *Nosokomeion* 6, no. 1–2 (Jan./Apr. 1935): 104–6.

———. "Sound Absorption, Insulation and Air Control: An Important Trio." *Modern Hospital* 45, no. 4 (Oct. 1935): 88–92.

———. "St. Luke's Hospital, Jacksonville, Florida." *Modern Hospital* 3, no. 4 (Oct. 1914): 218–27.

———. "The Surgical Unit." *Modern Hospital* 1, no. 1 (Sept. 1913): 18–21.

———. "This Hospital to Be Continued." *Modern Hospital* 53, no. 4 (Oct. 1939): 84–87.

———. "The Transformation of a Dwelling House into a Hospital." *Architect and Engineer of California* 52, no. 3 (Mar. 1918): 73–78.

———. "The Transformation of a Dwelling House into a Hospital." *Modern Hospital* 10, no. 2 (Feb. 1918): 75–79.

———. "The Trend in Hospital Construction on the North American Continent." *Canadian Hospital* 9, no. 1 (Jan. 1932): 24–32.

———. "The Ward and Operating Units of the General Hospital." *Modern Hospital* 1, no. 1 (Sept. 1913): 39–41.

———. "What the Past Fifteen Years Have Taught Us in Hospital Construction and Design." *American Architect* 132, no. 2534 (5 Dec. 1927): 701–8.

———. "Will the Consolidated Hospital Supplant the Small Hospital?" *Modern Hospital* 33, no. 2 (Aug. 1929): 92–94.

———. "A World-wide Comment on Hospital Construction." *Nosokomeion* 10, no. 4 (1939): 271–73.

———, and Charles Butler. "Our Overseas Hospitals." *American Architect* 113, no. 2216 (12 June 1918): 785–800.

———, and H. E. Webster. "Ross Pavilion of the Royal Victoria Hospital." *Modern Hospital* 12, no. 5 (May 1919): 311–15.

Stevens, Rosemary. *In Sickness and in Wealth: American Hospitals in the Twentieth Century.* New York: Basic, 1989.

Stevenson, Christine. "Medicine and Architecture." In *Companion Encyclopedia of the History of Medicine,* edited by W. F. Bynum and Roy Porter, 2:1495–1519. London: Routledge, 1993.

Stewart, Lee. *It's Up to You: Women at UBC in the Early Years.* Vancouver: UBC Press, 1990.

"St. Justine's Hospital, Montreal." *Construction* 21 (Mar. 1928): 87.

Stokes, Charles W. *Here and There in Montreal and the Island of Montreal.* Toronto: Musson, 1924.

"Student Nurses' Residence, Royal Victoria Hospital, Barrie, Ontario." *Journal (Royal Architectural Institute of Canada)* (Oct. 1952): 293.

Taylor, Jeremy. *The Architect and the Pavilion Hospital: Dialogue and Design Creativity in England, 1850–1914.* London: Leicester University Press, 1997.

Terry, Neville. *The Royal Vic: The Story of Montreal's Royal Victoria Hospital, 1894–1994.* Montreal: McGill-Queen's University Press, 1994.

"This Telephone Switchboard is Capable of Serving a City of 20.000." *Canadian Hospital* 7, no. 5 (May 1930): 46, 56.

Thompson, John D., and Grace Goldin. *The Hospital: A Social and Architectural History.* New Haven, Conn.: Yale University Press, 1975.

"A Three and a Half Million Dollar Hospital." *Contract Record and Engineering Review* 38, no. 53 (31 Dec. 1924): 1317–19.

Tomes, Nancy. *The Gospel of Germs: Men, Women, and the Microbe in American Life.* Cambridge, Mass.: Harvard University Press, 1998.

"Toronto Hospital for Sick Children, Toronto." *Construction* 7, no. 10 (Oct. 1914): 378–81.

Townley, Fred L. "The Planning of Nurses' Homes." *Journal (Royal Architectural Institute of Canada)* (Aug. 1944): 169–70.

Upton, Dell. *Architecture in the United States.* Oxford: Oxford University Press, 1998.

———. *Holy Things and Profane: Anglican Parish Churches in Colonial Virginia.* New York and Cambridge, Mass.: Architectural History Foundation and MIT Press, 1986.

"Urges Elaborate Hospitals." *Hospital World* 6 (Nov. 1914): 227–28.

Van Slyck, Abigail A. *Free to All: Carnegie Libraries and American Culture, 1890–1920*. Chicago: University of Chicago Press, 1995.

———. "The Lady and the Library Loafer: Gender and Public Space in Victorian America." *Winterthur Portfolio* 31, no. 4 (Winter 1996): 221–42.

———. *A Manufactured Wilderness: Summer Camps and the Shaping of American Youth, 1890–1960*. Minneapolis: University of Minnesota Press, 2006.

Verderber, Stephen, and David J. Fine. *Healthcare Architecture in an Era of Radical Transformation*. New Haven, Conn.: Yale University Press, 2000.

Vicinus, Martha. *Independent Women: Work and Community for Single Women 1850–1920*. Chicago: University of Chicago Press, 1985.

"The Victoria Hospital, Montreal." *Canadian Architect and Builder* (May 1889): 52.

Vogel, Morris J. *The Invention of the Modern Hospital: Boston, 1870–1930*. Chicago: University of Chicago Press, 1980.

Wagg, Susan. *Percy Erskine Nobbs: Architect, Artist, Craftsman*. Montreal: McCord Museum, 1982.

Walsh, William Henry, and Edgar Martin. "Hospital Planning and Construction." *Transactions of the AHA* 34 (1932): 284–93.

Wangensteen, Owen H., and Sarah D. Wangensteen. *The Rise of Surgery: From Empiric Craft to Scientific Discipline*. Minneapolis: University of Minnesota Press, 1978.

Weiner, Deborah. *Architecture and Social Reform in Late-Victorian London*. Manchester: Manchester University Press, 1994.

Weir, George. *Survey of Nursing Education in Canada*. Toronto: University of Toronto Press, 1932.

"Well Known Hospital Architects Form Partnership." *Canadian Hospital* (May 1932): 29.

Withey, Henry F. *Biographical Dictionary of American Architects*. Los Angeles: New Age, 1956.

Wright, Gwendolyn. *Moralism and the Model Home: Domestic Architecture and Cultural Conflict In Chicago, 1873–1913*. Chicago: University of Chicago Press, 1980.

York, Edward, and Philip Sawyer. *Specifications for a Hospital*. New York: Pencil Points, 1927.

Illustration Credits

Courtesy of the Alumnae Association of the Royal Victoria Hospital Training School for Nurses: 1.7, 3.6, 3.9.

Courtesy of the Archives of Ontario, Toronto, Arthur Heeny *fonds* C27 series C-1: 2.8, 2.12, 2.13, 2.15, 5.3, 5.5, 5.16.

Courtesy of the author: 1.17, 2.18, 5.2.

Courtesy of the Canadian Centre for Architecture: 3.11.

Courtesy of François-Xavier Caron: 3.8.

Courtesy of CHU Ste-Justine: 2.20.

Courtesy of City of Ottawa Archives, Ottawa Civic Hospital *fonds*, CA-2469 and CA-2453: 5.9, 5.13.

Courtesy of Hôpital Notre-Dame (Centre hospitalier de l'Université de Montréal): I.1.

Courtesy of the John Bland Canadian Architecture Collection, McGill University Library: 1.14, 1.15, 1.16, 1.18, 3.3, 3.4.

Courtesy of Céline Lemercier: 5.1.

Courtesy of the McCord Museum, Montreal: 1.4 (MP-000.1767), 1.6 (II-105911.0), 1.10 (VIEW-2733), 1.11 (VIEW-2735), 1.12 (II-73328), 1.13 (VIEW-2818), 2.16 (II-105910).

Courtesy of the McGill University Archives: 3.5, 3.12, 5.8.

Courtesy of Montreal Children's Hospital (McGill University Health Centre): 2.23, 2.24, 2.26, 2.27, 2.29, 2.30.

Courtesy of Christian Paquin: 1.2.

Courtesy of Rare Books and Special Collections Division, McGill University Library: 1.1.

Courtesy of Royal British Columbia Museum, B-09491: 4.10.

Courtesy of the Royal Victoria Hospital (McGill University Health Center): 1.5, 1.8, 1.19, 2.17, 3.2, 3.7, 5.14, 5.15.

Courtesy of the School of Architecture Slide Library, McGill University: 1.3.

Index

Annmarie Adams is William C. Macdonald Professor at the School of Architecture at McGill University in Montreal. She is author of *Architecture in the Family Way: Doctors, Houses, and Women, 1870–1900* and coauthor of *Designing Women: Gender and the Architectural Profession.*